It's easy to get lost in the cancer world

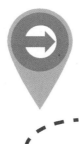

Let
**NCCN Guidelines
for Patients®
be your guide**

✓ Step-by-step guides to the cancer care options likely to have the best results

✓ Based on treatment guidelines used by health care providers worldwide

✓ Designed to help you discuss cancer treatment with your doctors

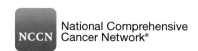
National Comprehensive
Cancer Network®

NCCN Guidelines for Patients® are developed by the National Comprehensive Cancer Network® (NCCN®)

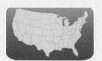

NCCN

✓ An alliance of leading cancer centers across the United States devoted to patient care, research, and education

Cancer centers that are part of NCCN:
NCCN.org/cancercenters

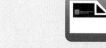

NCCN Clinical Practice Guidelines in Oncology (NCCN Guidelines®)

✓ Developed by doctors from NCCN cancer centers using the latest research and years of experience

✓ For providers of cancer care all over the world

✓ Expert recommendations for cancer screening, diagnosis, and treatment

Free online at
NCCN.org/guidelines

NCCN Guidelines for Patients

✓ Present information from the NCCN Guidelines in an easy-to-learn format

✓ For people with cancer and those who support them

✓ Explain the cancer care options likely to have the best results

Free online at
NCCN.org/patientguidelines

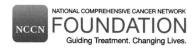
NATIONAL COMPREHENSIVE CANCER NETWORK
FOUNDATION
Guiding Treatment. Changing Lives.

and supported by funding from NCCN Foundation®

These NCCN Guidelines for Patients are based on the NCCN Guidelines® for Ovarian Cancer, Version 1.2021 — February 26, 2021.

NCCN Foundation seeks to support the millions of patients and their families affected by a cancer diagnosis by funding and distributing NCCN Guidelines for Patients. NCCN Foundation is also committed to advancing cancer treatment by funding the nation's promising doctors at the center of innovation in cancer research. For more details and the full library of patient and caregiver resources, visit NCCN.org/patients.

National Comprehensive Cancer Network (NCCN) / NCCN Foundation
3025 Chemical Road, Suite 100
Plymouth Meeting, PA 19462
215.690.0300

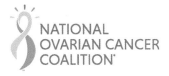

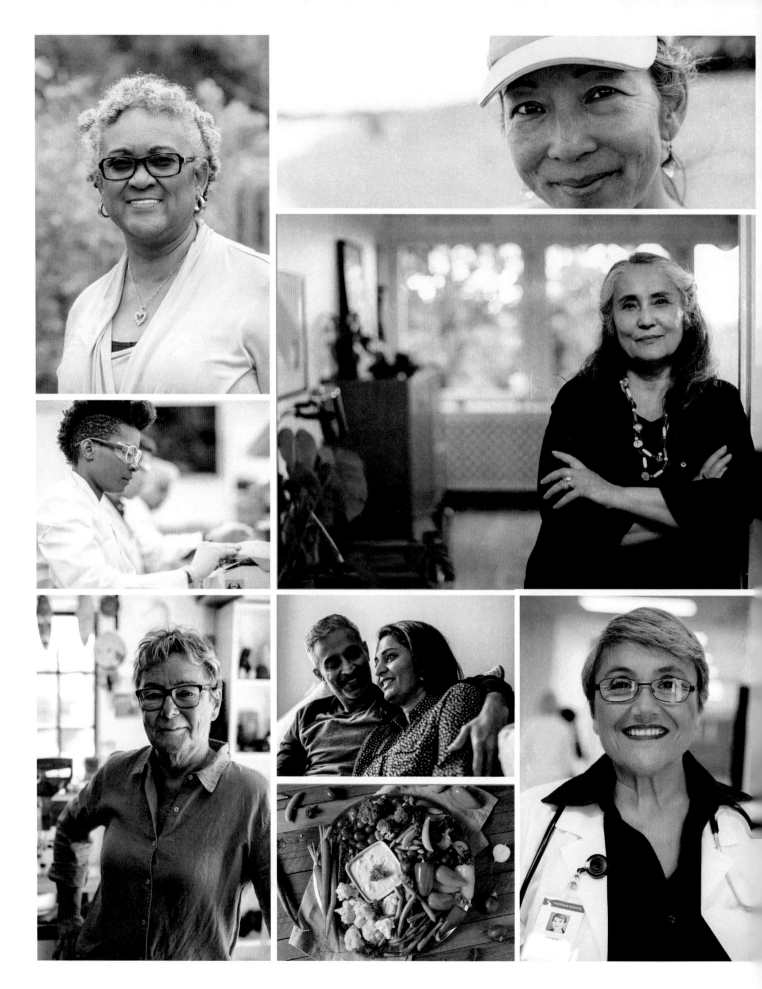

Contents

1
Ovarian cancer basics

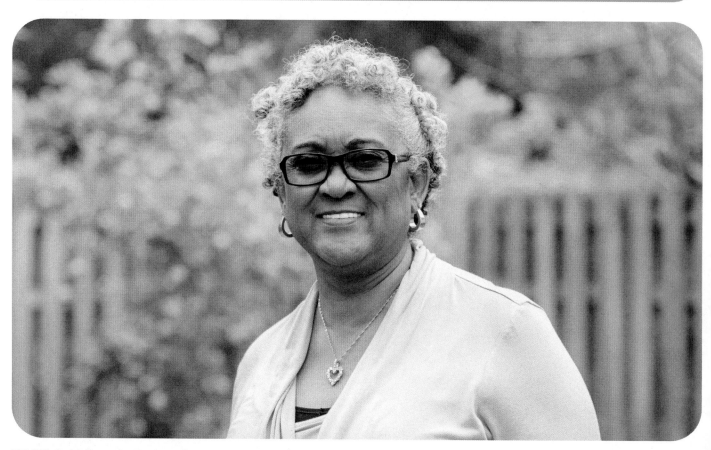

Most ovarian cancers start in the layer of tissue surrounding the ovaries, called the epithelium. The information in this patient guide applies to the most common types of epithelial ovarian cancer.

The ovaries

The ovaries are a pair of organs that are part of the female reproductive system. The reproductive system is the group of organs that work together for the purpose of sexual reproduction. In addition to the ovaries, this system includes the fallopian tubes, uterus, cervix, and vagina.

Each ovary is about the size and shape of a grape. The ovaries are located in the pelvis— the area below the belly (abdomen) and between the hip bones. One ovary is on the left side of the uterus and one is on the right. Each ovary is connected to the uterus by a long, thin tube called a fallopian tube.

The ovaries make eggs for sexual reproduction. They also make hormones that affect breast growth, body shape, and the menstrual cycle. Eggs pass out of the ovary and travel through the attached fallopian tube into the uterus. The uterus is where an unborn baby grows and develops during pregnancy. It is also called the womb. The uterus and at least one ovary are needed for menstruation and pregnancy.

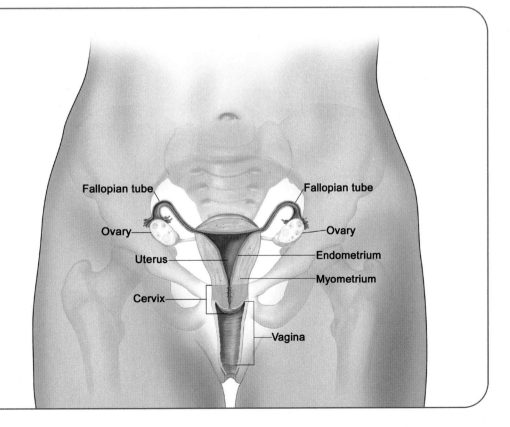

The reproductive system

The reproductive system is a group of organs that work together for the purpose of sexual reproduction. In addition to the ovaries, this system includes the fallopian tubes, uterus, cervix, and vagina.

Fallopian tube · Fallopian tube · Ovary · Ovary · Uterus · Endometrium · Myometrium · Cervix · Vagina

Types of ovarian cancer

As discussed later in this guide, surgery is the recommended first treatment for most ovarian cancers when possible. The tumor and other tissue removed during surgery are sent to an expert in testing cells to find disease, called a pathologist. The pathologist determines the specific type of ovarian cancer by examining the cancerous tissue.

The pathologist also determines the cancer grade, which is different than the cancer stage. The cancer grade is a rating of how fast the cancer is expected to grow and spread. It is based on how abnormal the cancer cells look under a microscope. High-grade cancers grow and spread more quickly than low-grade cancers.

The most common type of ovarian cancer is called epithelial ovarian cancer. It starts in the layer of tissue surrounding the ovaries (the epithelium). There are more than 5 different subtypes of epithelial ovarian cancer. Some are much more common than others. The information in this patient guide applies to the most common forms of epithelial ovarian cancer, listed below:

- High-grade (grade 2 or 3) serous carcinoma

- High-grade (grade 2 or 3) endometrioid carcinoma

Less common ovarian cancers

Other, rare types of ovarian cancer are referred to as less common ovarian cancers (LCOCs) or less common ovarian histologies (LCOHs). For your reference, these less common types of ovarian cancer are listed below. Treatment of these ovarian cancers is beyond the scope of this guide.

Less common **epithelial** ovarian cancers:

- Low-grade serous carcinoma

- Grade 1 endometrioid carcinoma

- Carcinosarcoma (malignant mixed Mullerian tumors [MMMTs] of the ovary)

- Clear cell carcinoma

- Mucinous carcinoma

- Low malignant potential (LMP) tumors (also known as borderline epithelial tumors)

Less common **non-epithelial** ovarian cancers:

- Malignant sex-cord stromal tumors

- Malignant germ cell tumors

Cancer cells

Cancer cells act differently than normal cells in three key ways. First, cancer cells grow without control. Unlike normal cells, cancer cells make new cells that are not needed and do not die when they should. The cancer cells build up to form a primary tumor.

Second, cancer cells can grow into (invade) other tissues. This is called invasion. Normal cells do not do this. Over time, the primary tumor can grow large and invade tissues outside the ovary. Ovarian cancer often invades the fallopian tubes and uterus.

Third, unlike normal cells, cancer cells can spread to other parts of the body. This process is called metastasis. Ovarian cancer cells can break off (shed) from the primary tumor to form new tumors on the surface of nearby organs and tissues. These are called "implants" or "seeds." Implants that grow into supporting tissues of nearby organs are called invasive implants.

Cancer cells can also spread through blood or lymph vessels. Lymph is a clear fluid made of white blood cells that help fight germs. It travels in small tubes (vessels) to lymph nodes. Lymph nodes are small groups of disease-fighting cells that remove germs from lymph. Lymph vessels and nodes are found all over the body.

Testing for ovarian cancer

Your doctor may suspect ovarian cancer if you have certain symptoms. Symptoms are changes in the body that you can feel or notice. Unfortunately, ovarian cancer may not cause symptoms until the tumor has grown very large or has spread. The most common symptoms include:

> Feeling bloated

> Heartburn and indigestion

> Pain in the pelvis or belly (abdomen)

> Trouble eating or feeling full fast (early satiety)

> Feeling the need to urinate often or urgently

These symptoms can also be caused by other common health conditions. Ovarian cancer is more likely to be the cause of these symptoms if they are new (began less than a year ago), frequent (occurring more than 12 days each month), or becoming more severe over time.

Other symptoms may develop if the mass is large or if fluid builds up in your abdomen. Your doctor may be able to feel a mass by doing a pelvic or abdominal exam (described on the following page). The buildup of fluid is called ascites and this may cause swelling of the abdomen. If your doctor suspects ovarian cancer based on your symptoms, you will have testing as described in this chapter.

Some tests are done at the initial visit, while others are done soon after a diagnosis is made. It is helpful to ask your doctor which tests you will have and when you can expect the results. The results of certain tests and evaluations described in this chapter provide important information needed to plan treatment. Your doctor uses the results of these initial tests to:

> **Determine the clinical (pre-surgery) stage.** The clinical stage provides a "best guess" of how far the cancer has spread. It is a best guess because surgery is needed in order to know exactly how much cancer is in the body.

> **Determine whether you are a good candidate for surgery.** Having surgery first may not be an option based on the size and location of the tumor. Having surgery first may also not be a good option for those who are elderly, frail, have trouble doing daily activities, or who have other serious health conditions. If your doctor decides that having surgery first isn't a good choice for you, see *If surgery first is not an option* on page 42. Otherwise, keep reading.

Biopsy

To confirm if you have ovarian cancer, a sample of tissue must be removed from your body for testing. This is called a biopsy. Doctors test tumor tissue to check for cancer cells and to look at the features of the cancer cells. Most often, the biopsy is done during surgery to remove ovarian cancer.

For some patients a biopsy may be done before treatment to help make the diagnosis of ovarian cancer prior to surgery or planned treatment. This may be done if the cancer has spread too much to be removed by initial surgery. In such cases, a fine-needle aspiration (FNA) biopsy or paracentesis may be used. An FNA biopsy uses a very thin needle to remove a small sample of tissue from the tumor. For paracentesis, a long, thin needle is inserted through the skin of the belly (abdomen) to remove a sample of fluid.

The biopsy samples will be sent to a pathologist for testing. A pathologist is a doctor who is an expert in testing cells to find disease. The pathologist will view the samples with a microscope to look for cancer cells. If the cells are cancerous, the pathologist will assess the features of the cancer cells.

Review of tumor tissue

Sometimes ovarian cancer is confirmed by a prior surgery or biopsy performed by another doctor. In this case, your doctors will need to review all of the prior results. This includes results of the surgery, biopsy, and tests of tissue that was removed. A pathologist will examine the tumor tissue with a microscope to make sure it is ovarian cancer. Your doctors will also want to know if the surgery left any cancer in your body. All of this will help your current doctors plan treatment done during and after treatment to check treatment results.

Abdominal and pelvic exam

Your doctor will do a physical exam of your belly (abdomen) and pelvis—the area between your hip bones. This is called an abdominal and pelvic exam. For the abdominal exam, your doctor will feel different parts of your belly. This is to see if organs are of normal size, are soft or hard, or cause pain when touched. Your doctor will also feel for signs of fluid buildup, called ascites. Ascites may be found in the belly area or around the ovaries.

During the pelvic exam, your doctor will feel for abnormal changes in the size, shape, or position of your ovaries and uterus. A special widening instrument will be used to view your vagina and cervix. A sample of cells may be removed for testing. This is known as a Pap test.

Imaging tests

Imaging tests take pictures of the inside of your body. Doctors use imaging tests to check if there is a tumor in your ovaries. The pictures can show the tumor size, shape, and location. They can also show if the cancer has spread beyond your ovaries. Different types of imaging tests are used to look for ovarian cancer, plan treatment, and check treatment results.

Before the test, you may be asked to stop eating or drinking for a few hours. You may also need to remove metal objects from your body. The types of imaging tests used for ovarian cancer are described next.

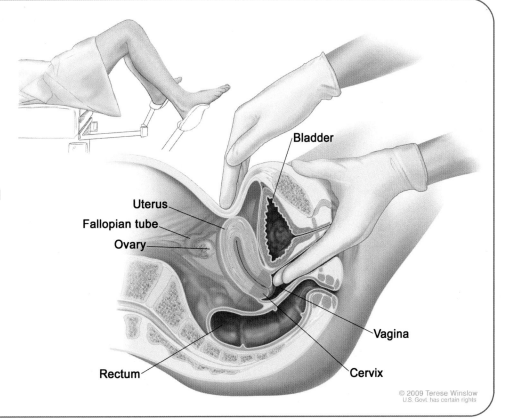

Pelvic exam

During a pelvic exam, your doctor will feel for abnormal changes in the size, shape, or position of your ovaries and uterus. A special widening instrument will be used to view your vagina and cervix.

Bladder, Uterus, Fallopian tube, Ovary, Rectum, Vagina, Cervix

© 2009 Terese Winslow
U.S. Govt. has certain rights

Ultrasound

Ultrasound is a test that uses sound waves to make pictures of the inside of the body. It is often the first imaging test given to look for ovarian cancer. Ultrasound is good at showing the size, shape, and location of the ovaries, fallopian tubes, uterus, and nearby tissues. It can also show if there is a mass in the ovary and whether the mass is solid or filled with fluid.

A hand-held device called an ultrasound probe is used. The probe sends out sound waves that bounce off organs and tissues to make echoes. The probe also picks up the echoes. A computer uses the echoes to make a picture that is shown on a screen. There are two types of ultrasounds that may be used to look for ovarian cancer: transabdominal ultrasound and transvaginal ultrasound.

For a transabdominal ultrasound, a gel will be spread on your stomach (abdomen) and the area between your hip bones (pelvis). The gel helps to make the pictures clearer. Your doctor will place the probe on your skin and guide it back and forth in the gel.

For a transvaginal ultrasound, your doctor will insert the probe into your vagina. This may help the doctor see your ovaries more clearly. Ultrasounds are generally painless, but you may feel some discomfort when the probe is inserted.

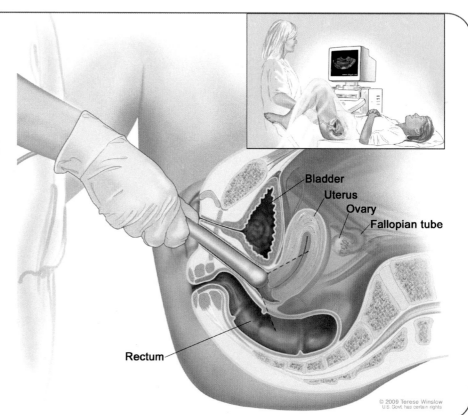

Transvaginal ultrasound

Ultrasound uses sound waves to make pictures of the inside of the body. For a transvaginal ultrasound, a probe is inserted into the vagina. Ultrasounds are generally painless, but you may feel some discomfort when the probe is inserted.

Bladder
Uterus
Ovary
Fallopian tube
Rectum

© 2009 Terese Winslow
U.S. Govt. has certain rights

Computed tomography (CT)

A CT scan uses x-rays to take many pictures of areas inside of the body from different angles. All of the x-ray pictures are combined to make one detailed picture of the body part.

CT scans of your chest, abdomen, and/or pelvis may be given along with other initial tests to look for ovarian cancer. This type of scan is good at showing if the cancer has spread outside of the ovaries. But, it is not good at showing small tumors. A CT scan may also show if nearby lymph nodes are bigger than normal, which can be a sign of cancer spread.

A substance called contrast will be used to make the pictures clearer. Before the CT scan, you will be asked to drink a large glass of oral contrast. A contrast agent will also be injected into your vein. This is referred to as intravenous ("IV") contrast. It may cause you to feel flushed or get hives. Rarely, serious allergic reactions occur. Tell your doctors if you have had bad (allergic) reactions to IV contrast in the past.

A CT scan machine is large and has a tunnel in the middle. During the scan, you will lie face up on a table that moves through the tunnel. The scanner will rotate an x-ray beam around you to take pictures from many angles. You may hear buzzing, clicking, or whirring sounds during this time. A computer will combine all the x-ray pictures into one detailed picture.

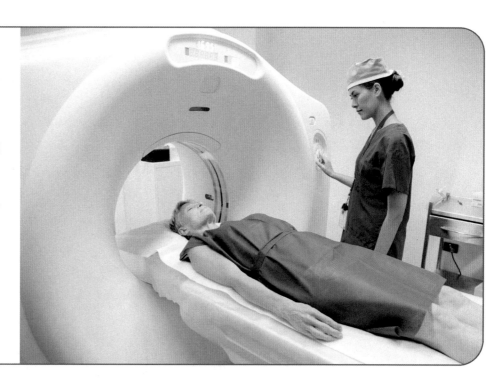

CT scan

A CT scan is a more detailed kind of x-ray. It takes a lot of pictures, or images, from different angles. A computer then combines the images to make 3-D pictures.

In some cases, CT may be combined with positron emission tomography (PET). A PET scan shows how your cells are using a simple form of sugar. To create pictures, a sugar radiotracer first needs to be put into your body with an injection into a vein. The radiotracer emits a small amount of energy that is detected by the machine that takes pictures. Active cancer cells use sugar faster than normal cells. Thus, cancer cells look brighter in the pictures. PET is very good at showing small groups of cancer cells. This test may also be useful for showing if ovarian cancer has spread.

Magnetic resonance imaging (MRI)

An MRI scan uses radio waves and powerful magnets to take pictures of the inside of the body. It does not use x-rays. This type of scan is good at showing the spine and soft tissues. An MRI scan of your abdomen and pelvis may be used to look for ovarian cancer if the ultrasound was unclear. An MRI scan of your chest may

be used to look for signs of cancer spread. This test may also be used to check treatment results and to assess for cancer spread to other parts of the body.

Getting an MRI scan is similar to getting a CT scan. But, MRI scans take longer to complete. The full exam can take an hour or more. For the scan, you will need to lie on a table that moves through a large tunnel in the scanning machine. The scan may cause your body to feel a bit warm. Like a CT scan, a contrast agent will be used to make the pictures clearer.

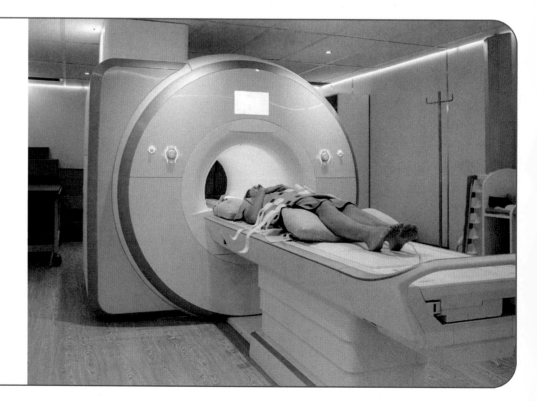

MRI machine

MRI makes pictures of areas inside the body without using radiation.

Chest x-ray

An x-ray uses small amounts of radiation to make pictures of organs and tissues inside the body. A tumor changes the way radiation is absorbed and will show up on the x-ray picture. A chest x-ray can be used to show if cancer has spread to your lungs. This test may be given with other initial tests when ovarian cancer is first suspected or found. It may also be given after treatment to check treatment results. A chest x-ray is painless and takes about 20 minutes to complete.

Family history and genetic testing

Ovarian cancer most often occurs for unknown reasons. However, about 15 out of 100 ovarian cancers are due to changes (mutations) in genes that are passed down from a parent to a child. This is called hereditary ovarian cancer.

Hereditary ovarian cancer is most often caused by mutations in 1 of 2 genes: breast cancer gene 1 (*BRCA1*) or breast cancer gene 2 (*BRCA2*). A *BRCA* mutation increases the risk of developing ovarian, breast, and some other cancers. Everyone has *BRCA1* and *BRCA2* genes. When working properly, they are helpful and prevent abnormal cell growth by repairing damaged cells.

Another cause of hereditary ovarian cancer is Lynch syndrome, also known as hereditary nonpolyposis colorectal cancer (HNPCC) syndrome. Lynch syndrome is the most common cause of hereditary colon cancer, but can also cause ovarian and other cancers.

Ovarian cancer associated with a *BRCA* mutation or Lynch syndrome usually starts at a younger age than non-hereditary ovarian cancer. Using your age, medical history, and family history, your doctor will assess how likely you are to have hereditary ovarian cancer.

Genetic testing can tell if you have a mutation in the *BRCA* genes, or in other genes that play a role in hereditary cancer. If initial treatment works well, *BRCA* status (whether you have a *BRCA* mutation) plays an important role in guiding decisions about maintenance therapy. Maintenance therapy is discussed in more detail later in this guide.

Genetic counseling is recommended for everyone diagnosed with ovarian cancer. Genetic counseling is a discussion with a health expert, typically a genetic counselor, about the risk for a disease caused by changes in genes. A genetic counselor has special training to help patients understand changes in genes that are related to disease. The genetic counselor can tell you more about how likely you are to have hereditary ovarian cancer, and may suggest genetic testing to look for changes in genes that increase the chances of developing ovarian cancer.

More information on *BRCA* mutations is provided in the *Tumor biomarker testing* section on page 17.

Nutritional and digestive tract health

While taking your medical and family history, your doctor may also ask about your diet and eating habits. Symptoms of ovarian cancer include bloating, pain in the pelvis or abdomen, difficulty eating, and feeling full quickly. These symptoms can lead to changes in eating habits, which can affect your overall health and nutrition level. If you are eating less in general, or not eating enough healthy foods, you may not be getting enough nutrients. A lack of nutrition can have an impact on the success of surgery and other treatment outcomes, especially in older patients. If you need help with keeping a healthy diet or have questions about your diet, ask your doctor for a referral to a registered dietitian.

In some cases, your doctor may want to evaluate your gastrointestinal (GI) tract using an imaging test. The GI tract is made of the organs that food passes through when you eat. This includes your stomach, small intestine, large intestine, and rectum. A GI evaluation may be used in certain cases to check for signs of cancer spread. It can help identify or rule out other cancers.

This imaging test uses a scope to see inside your GI tract. A scope is a long, thin tube that can be guided into your body, often through the mouth, anus, or a surgical cut. One end of the scope has a small light and camera lens to see inside your body. At the other end of the scope is an eyepiece that your doctor looks through to see the pictures shown by the camera.

Blood tests

Doctors test blood to look for signs of disease and to assess your general health. The following tests are not used to diagnose ovarian cancer, but abnormal results may signal health problems.

A **complete blood count (CBC)** measures the number of red blood cells, white blood cells, and platelets in a sample of blood. Your doctor will want to know if you have enough red blood cells to carry oxygen throughout your body, white blood cells to fight infections, and platelets to control bleeding. Your blood counts may be abnormal—too low or too high—because of cancer or other health problems.

A **blood chemistry profile** measures the levels of different chemicals in your blood. Chemicals in your blood come from your liver, bones, and other organs and tissues. Doctors use this test to assess the health of organs such as your liver and kidneys. Abnormal blood chemistry levels—too high or too low—may be a sign that an organ isn't working well. Abnormal levels may also be caused by the spread of cancer or by other diseases. Your doctor will consider your health and look at the whole profile when it comes to blood test results.

The liver is an organ that does many important jobs, such as remove toxins from your blood. **Liver function tests** measure chemicals that are made or processed by the liver. Levels that are too high or low may be a sign of liver damage or cancer spread. Liver function tests are often done along with a blood chemistry profile.

Tumor marker blood tests

A tumor marker is a substance found in body tissue or fluid that may be a sign of cancer. When considered with other information, tumor markers can help diagnose ovarian cancer. They can also be used to monitor response to treatment.

CA-125 (cancer antigen-125) is the most commonly used tumor marker test for ovarian cancer. CA-125 is a protein made by normal cells and ovarian cancer cells. High levels of CA-125 in the blood may be a sign of certain cancers, including ovarian cancer.

A CA-125 test measures the amount of CA-125 in the blood. This test alone cannot diagnose ovarian cancer. This is because there are non-cancerous conditions that can raise your CA-125 level. Also, some ovarian cancers do not cause an elevated CA-125 level. But, CA-125 testing may be done along with other initial tests if your doctor suspects ovarian cancer. It may also be done during and after treatment to check treatment results.

Your blood may also be tested for the following tumor markers. These tumor markers may be found in higher-than-normal amounts in people with rare ovarian tumor types, called less common ovarian cancers (LCOCs).

> - Inhibin (typically inhibin A and inhibin B)
> - Beta-human chorionic gonadotropin (β-hCG)
> - Alpha-fetoprotein (AFP)
> - Lactate dehydrogenase (LDH)
> - Carcinoembryonic antigen (CEA)
> - CA 19-9

Tumor biomarker testing

Treatment options for patients with advanced ovarian cancer may include targeted therapy or immunotherapy. Like chemotherapy, these are medicines that work throughout the body to treat cancer. Unlike chemotherapy, these newer therapies are most effective at treating cancers with specific features, called biomarkers.

Biomarkers are specific features of cancer cells. Biomarkers can include proteins made in response to the cancer and changes (mutations) in the DNA of the cancer cells. Biomarker testing is used to learn whether your cancer has any targetable changes to help guide your treatment. If it does, targeted therapy or immunotherapy may be a treatment option if needed. The results of biomarker testing can also be used to determine whether you meet the criteria for joining certain clinical trials.

Testing for biomarker mutations involves analyzing a piece of tumor tissue in a laboratory or testing a sample of blood. Other names for biomarker testing include molecular testing, genomic testing, tumor gene testing, and mutation testing.

While everyone diagnosed with ovarian cancer should be tested for *BRCA* mutations, the timing and number of other biomarker tests can vary and are at the discretion of your doctor.

Some doctors choose to test for a number of biomarkers all at once early in the treatment process. Others may only test for *BRCA* early in the treatment process and wait to see if therapies that require specific biomarkers are needed.

BRCA and HRD

Everyone with suspected or confirmed ovarian cancer should have their tumor tested for mutations in the *BRCA1* and *BRCA2* genes, and other similar genes important in DNA repair. This is different than genetic testing of the blood for inherited ("germline") *BRCA* mutations. Mutations in the tumor itself are known as "somatic" (or simply "tumor") mutations.

A *BRCA* mutation is the most important biomarker used to plan ovarian cancer treatment. *BRCA* mutations are a form of homologous recombination deficiency (HRD). This means that if you have a *BRCA* mutation, your cancer is, by extension, homologous recombination deficient. You may also hear the term "HRD positive" used to describe homologous recombination deficient cancers.

However, you can also be HRD positive without a *BRCA* mutation. Other changes in your tumor's DNA can make it homologous recombination deficient. Your *BRCA* and HRD status are used to guide decisions about maintenance therapy after initial treatment. More information on maintenance therapy is provided in *Part 2: Treatment guide.*

MMR/MSI

In normal cells, a process called mismatch repair (MMR) fixes errors (mutations) that happen when the DNA divides and makes a copy of itself. If the MMR system isn't working right, errors build up and cause the DNA to become unstable. This is called microsatellite instability (MSI). There are two kinds of laboratory tests for this biomarker. Depending on the method used, an abnormal result is called either microsatellite instability high (MSI-H) or mismatch repair deficient

(dMMR). Both results mean the same thing. Pembrolizumab (Keytruda®) is an immunotherapy that may be used to target advanced or metastatic cancer that is MSI-H or dMMR.

Tumor mutational burden

The total number of mutations (changes) found in the DNA of cancer cells is known as the tumor mutational burden (TMB). A tumor with 10 or more mutations is referred to as tumor mutational burden-high (TMB-H). Pembrolizumab (Keytruda®) is an immunotherapy that may be used to target advanced or metastatic cancer that has a high number of mutations.

NTRK gene fusion

This biomarker is rare in ovarian cancer. In a tumor with a neurotrophin receptor kinase *(NTRK)* gene fusion, a piece of the *NTRK* gene and a piece of another gene fuse, or join. This activates the *NTRK* gene in a way that causes uncontrolled cell growth. Larotrectinib (Vitrakvi®) and entrectinib (Rozlytrek®) are targeted therapies that might be used to target advanced or metastatic cancer that is *NTRK* gene fusion-positive.

Cancer care plan

Your treatment team

Treating ovarian cancer may consist of a team of gynecologic oncologists and medical oncologists. NCCN experts recommend that a gynecologic oncologist should perform the initial surgery for ovarian cancer when possible. A gynecologic oncologist is an expert in surgery and chemotherapy for gynecologic cancers. Sometimes, a medical oncologist who is an expert in treating cancer with chemotherapy may administer treatment.

Your primary care physician (PCP) can also be a part of your team. Your PCP can help you express your feelings about treatments to the team. Treatment of other medical problems may be improved if your PCP is informed of your cancer care. In addition to doctors, you may receive care from nurses, social workers, and other health experts. Ask to have the names and contact information of your health care providers included in the treatment plan.

Cancer treatment

There is no single treatment practice that is best for all patients. There is often more than one treatment option, including clinical trials. Clinical trials study the safety and effectiveness of investigational treatments.

The treatment that you and your doctors agree on should be reported in the treatment plan. It is also important to note the goal of treatment and the chance of a good treatment outcome. All known side effects should be listed and the time required to treat them should be noted.

Your treatment plan may change because of new information. You may change your mind about treatment. Tests may find new results. How well the treatment is working may change. Any of these changes may require a new treatment plan.

Stress and symptom control

Cancer and its treatment can cause bothersome symptoms. The stress of having cancer can also cause symptoms. There are ways to treat many symptoms, so tell your treatment team about any that you have.

Feelings of anxiety and depression are common among people with cancer. At your cancer center, cancer navigators, social workers, and other experts can help. Help can include support groups, talk therapy, or medication. Some people also feel better by exercising, talking with loved ones, or relaxing.

You may be unemployed or miss work during treatment. Or, you may have too little or no health insurance. Talk to your treatment team about work, insurance, or money problems. They will include information in the treatment plan to help you manage your finances and medical costs.

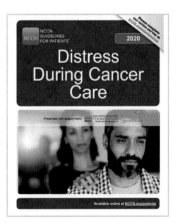

See the *NCCN Guidelines for Patients: Distress During Cancer Care* at NCCN.org/patientguidelines for more information.

Supportive care

Supportive care is treatment given to relieve the symptoms of cancer or the side effects of cancer treatment. It aims to relieve discomfort and improve quality of life. Supportive care may be given alone or in combination with cancer treatment.

Advance care planning

Talking with your doctor about your prognosis can help with treatment planning. If the cancer cannot be controlled or cured, a care plan for the end of life can be made. There are many benefits to advance care planning, including:

> Knowing what to expect

> Making the most of your time

> Lowering the stress of caregivers

> Having your wishes followed

> Having a better quality of life

> Getting good care

Advance care planning starts with an honest talk between you and your doctors. You don't have to know the exact details of your prognosis. Just having a general idea will help with planning. With this information, you can decide at what point you will want to stop chemotherapy or other treatments, if at all. You can also decide what treatments you will want for symptom relief, such as surgery or medicine.

Another part of the planning involves hospice care. Hospice care does not include treatment to fight the cancer but rather to reduce symptoms caused by cancer. Hospice care may be started because you aren't interested in more cancer treatment, no other cancer treatment is available, or because you may be too sick for cancer treatment.

Hospice care allows you to have the best quality of life possible. Care is given all day, every day of the week. You can choose to have hospice care at home or at a hospice center. One study found that patients and caregivers had a better quality of life when hospice care was started early.

An advance directive describes the treatment you'd want if you weren't able to make your wishes known. It also can name a person whom you'd want to make decisions for you. It is a legal paper that your doctors have to follow. It can reveal your wishes about life-sustaining machines, such as feeding tubes. It can also include your treatment wishes if your heart or lungs were to stop working. If you already have an advance directive, it may need to be updated to be legally valid.

Clinical trials

A clinical trial is a type of medical research study. After being developed and tested in a laboratory, potential new ways of fighting cancer need to be studied in people. If found to be safe and effective in a clinical trial, a drug, device, or treatment approach may be approved by the U.S. Food and Drug Administration (FDA).

Everyone with cancer should carefully consider all of the treatment options available for their cancer type, including standard treatments and clinical trials. Talk to your doctor about whether a clinical trial may make sense for you.

Phases

Most cancer clinical trials focus on treatment. Treatment trials are done in phases.

> - **Phase I** trials study the dose, safety, and side effects of an investigational drug or treatment approach. They also look for early signs that the drug or approach is helpful.

> - **Phase II** trials study how well the drug or approach works against a specific type of cancer.

> - **Phase III** trials test the drug or approach against a standard treatment. If the results are good, it may be approved by the FDA.

> - **Phase IV** trials study the long-term safety and benefit of an FDA-approved treatment.

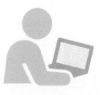

Finding a clinical trial

In the United States

NCCN Cancer Centers
NCCN.org/cancercenters

The National Cancer Institute (NCI)
cancer.gov/about-cancer/treatment/clinical-trials/search

Worldwide

The U.S. National Library of Medicine (NLM)
clinicaltrials.gov/

Need help finding a clinical trial?
NCI's Cancer Information Service (CIS)
1.800.4.CANCER (1.800.422.6237)
cancer.gov/contact

Who can enroll?

Every clinical trial has rules for joining, called eligibility criteria. The rules may be about age, cancer type and stage, treatment history, or general health. These requirements ensure that participants are alike in specific ways and that the trial is as safe as possible for the participants.

Informed consent

Clinical trials are managed by a group of experts called a research team. The research team will review the study with you in detail, including its purpose and the risks and benefits of joining. All of this information is also provided in an informed consent form. Read the form carefully and ask questions before signing it. Take time to discuss with family, friends, or others you trust. Keep in mind that you can leave and seek treatment outside of the clinical trial at any time.

Start the conversation

Don't wait for your doctor to bring up clinical trials. Start the conversation and learn about all of your treatment options. If you find a study that you may be eligible for, ask your treatment team if you meet the requirements. Try not to be discouraged if you cannot join. New clinical trials are always becoming available.

Frequently asked questions

There are many myths and misconceptions surrounding clinical trials. The possible benefits and risks are not well understood by many with cancer.

Will I get a placebo?

Placebos (inactive versions of real medicines) are almost never used alone in cancer clinical trials. It is common to receive either a placebo with a standard treatment, or a new drug with a standard treatment. You will be informed, verbally and in writing, if a placebo is part of a clinical trial before you enroll.

Do I have to pay to be in a clinical trial?

Rarely. It depends on the study, your health insurance, and the state in which you live. Your treatment team and the research team can help determine if you are responsible for any costs.

Key points

- The ovaries are a pair of organs that make eggs for sexual reproduction. They also make hormones.

- Ovarian cancer often starts in the cells that form the outer layer of tissue around the ovaries. This is called epithelial ovarian cancer.

- The most common epithelial ovarian tumor types are high-grade serous carcinoma and high-grade endometrioid carcinoma. These tumor types are the focus of this patient guide.

- Symptoms of ovarian cancer include bloating, heartburn, indigestion, pain in the belly or pelvis, trouble eating, and needing to urinate often or urgently.

- Testing for suspected ovarian cancer includes imaging tests, general blood tests, and tumor marker tests that are used to plan treatment for ovarian cancer.

- NCCN experts recommend genetic counseling for everyone diagnosed with ovarian cancer. Genetic counseling may help you decide whether to be tested for hereditary ovarian cancer.

- Hereditary ovarian cancer is most often caused by mutations in the *BRCA1* and *BRCA2* genes. Families with a history of Lynch syndrome may also be at risk for ovarian and other cancers.

- High levels of CA-125 in the blood may be a sign of ovarian cancer. A blood test for CA-125 may be done if your doctor suspects ovarian cancer. It may also be done during and after treatment to check treatment results.

- Biomarker testing looks for unique features or characteristics of a cancer, such as tumor mutations, that can help guide your treatment.

- Treating ovarian cancer takes a team of experts. Gynecologic oncologists and medical oncologists often work together to plan the best treatment for ovarian cancer.

- Your treatment plan should include a schedule of follow-up cancer tests, treatment of long-term side effects, and care of your general health.

- Clinical trials give people access to investigational treatments that may, in time, be approved by the FDA.

2
Treatment guide

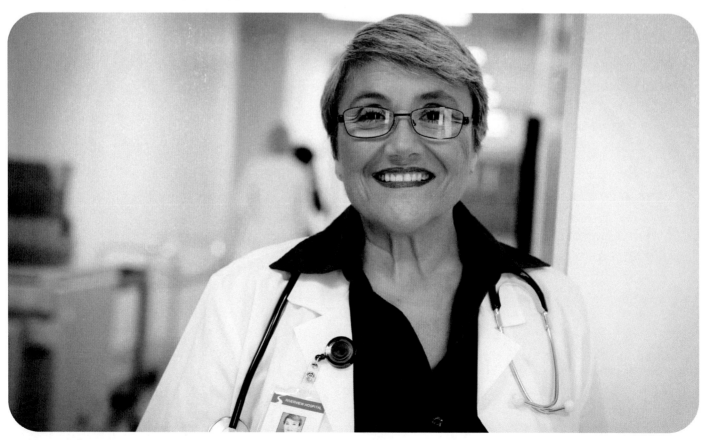

Surgery

Surgery is the recommended first treatment for all women with ovarian cancer who are willing and able to have it. If you cannot have surgery first, see page 42. Ovarian cancer surgery should be performed by a gynecologic oncologist. A gynecologic oncologist is a surgeon who is an expert in cancers that start in the female reproductive organs.

A main goal of surgery for ovarian cancer is to remove all or as much of the cancer from your body as possible. This involves removing the tumor as well as other organs and tissues where cancer cells have or might have spread. Another goal of surgery is to learn how far the cancer has spread. While testing before surgery can give your doctors an idea of how far the cancer may have spread, surgery is needed to know the true extent of the cancer.

Types of ovarian cancer surgery

The most commonly used surgery is actually two surgeries—hysterectomy and bilateral salpingo-oophorectomy (BSO). A hysterectomy is surgery to remove the uterus. When the cervix is removed in addition to the uterus, it is called a "total" or "complete" hysterectomy. A BSO removes both ovaries and both fallopian tubes. Pregnancy is not possible after a hysterectomy. Fertility-sparing surgery (described below) may be an option for some women with very early ovarian cancer that has not spread beyond the ovaries.

If cancer has spread outside the ovaries, your surgeon will attempt to remove all of the cancer that can be seen. This is called debulking or cytoreductive surgery. Debulking surgery removes as much cancer as possible. The extent of the surgery depends on how far the cancer has spread. It may remove all or part of nearby organs such as the liver, spleen, stomach, gallbladder, pancreas, intestines, appendix, and bladder. Lymph nodes that look abnormal or are larger than normal should also be removed if possible.

Fertility-sparing surgery

Women who have their uterus removed are not able to become pregnant. This can be difficult to accept for some younger women diagnosed with ovarian cancer. For these women, fertility-sparing surgery may be an option. In fertility-sparing surgery, one or both ovaries and fallopian tubes are removed, but the uterus is left in place. Surgery to remove one ovary and one fallopian tube is called a unilateral salpingo-oophorectomy (USO). USO is only an option if the cancer is only in one ovary. After a USO, you may still be able to become pregnant naturally if you haven't yet gone through menopause.

A BSO may be an option if the cancer is in both ovaries. A BSO removes both ovaries and both fallopian tubes. The uterus is not removed. While you cannot become pregnant naturally after a BSO, pregnancy may be possible using assisted reproductive approaches. One such approach is in vitro fertilization (IVF). In IVF, eggs are fertilized with sperm in a laboratory to create embryos. The embryos are then implanted into the uterus or frozen for future use. The eggs used for IVF may be yours (removed from your ovary before surgery) or donor eggs. Donor eggs are removed from women who have volunteered to go through hormone treatment to stimulate egg production in her ovaries.

Surgery methods

Most often, surgery is done using a laparotomy. A laparotomy is the most common and preferred method for ovarian cancer surgery. A laparotomy is a long surgical cut in the abdomen. It is often an up-and-down (vertical) cut from the top of the belly button down to the pelvic bone. This lets your doctor see the tumor and other organs and tissues in your abdomen and pelvis. NCCN experts recommend this method when surgical staging (described next) or debulking surgery is planned.

Less commonly, a minimally invasive type of surgery called laparoscopy may be used. Laparoscopy uses a few small cuts in the abdomen instead of one big one. Small tools are inserted through the cuts to perform the surgery. One of the tools is called a laparoscope. It is a long tube with a light and camera at the end. The camera lets your doctor see the ovaries and other tissues in the abdomen. The other tools are used to remove tissue.

Laparoscopy may be used in select cases, such as when cancer is only in the ovaries. It is rarely used when cancer has spread outside the ovaries. This surgery should only be done by a gynecologic oncologist experienced in this method.

Surgical staging

Regardless of the type of surgery you have, surgical staging should be performed. Surgical staging involves taking samples during surgery from organs and tissues where ovarian cancer often spreads. The samples are tested for cancer cells. Your surgeon will also take samples from nearby tissues where it looks like cancer has not spread. This is done to check for cancer cells that have spread outside the ovaries or pelvis and can only be seen with a microscope. These are called microscopic metastases.

Some or all of the omentum and nearby lymph nodes will be removed. The omentum is the fatty layer of tissue that covers organs in the belly (abdomen). Surgery to remove the omentum is called an omentectomy. Surgery to remove nearby lymph nodes is called a lymph node dissection.

Which surgical staging procedures you will have and the number of samples taken depends on how far your doctors think the cancer has spread. Samples may be taken from the following sites:

> Nearby lymph nodes – groups of disease-fighting cells

> Pelvis – the area below the belly (abdomen) between the hip bones

> Abdomen – the belly area between the chest and pelvis

> Diaphragm – the muscles below the ribs that help a person breathe

> Omentum – the layer of fatty tissue covering organs in the abdomen

> Peritoneum – the tissue that lines the inside of the abdomen and pelvis and covers most organs in this space

> Ascites – abnormal fluid buildup in the abdomen

If you do not have ascites, your doctor may "wash" the space inside your belly (peritoneal cavity) with a special liquid. This is called a peritoneal washing. Samples of the liquid will then be tested for cancer cells.

Surgical staging is the most complete and accurate way to stage ovarian cancer. The pathologic (post-surgery) stage is based on the results of surgery and tests of tissue removed during surgery. The pathologic stage provides the most accurate picture of how far the cancer has spread. The stages of ovarian cancer are explained on page 29.

Preparing for surgery

Your treatment team will give you instructions on how to prepare for your surgery. You may be asked to stop taking some medicines for a short time. You also should not eat or drink after midnight the night before the surgery.

On the day of your surgery, you will be given medicine to put you into a deep sleep so you won't feel pain. This is called general anesthesia. Surgery may take 3 or more hours to complete. More or less time may be needed depending on how much tissue is removed.

After the surgery, you will need to stay in the hospital for a few days or weeks to recover. You may feel some pain and tenderness in your belly and pelvis. This may last for a few days or weeks. You may be able to return to normal

activities in a few weeks. The time it takes to fully recover varies from person to person. It also varies depending on the extent of the surgery.

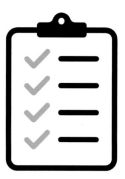

We want your feedback!

Our goal is to provide helpful and easy-to-understand information on cancer.

Take our survey to let us know what we got right and what we could do better:

NCCN.org/patients/feedback

Risks and side effects of surgery

With any type of surgery, there are some health risks and side effects. A side effect is a problem that occurs when treatment affects healthy tissues or organs. Common side effects of any surgery include pain, swelling, and scars. But, the side effects of surgery can differ between people. They also differ based on the type and extent of surgery.

Some common side effects of surgery for ovarian cancer include leg swelling, trouble urinating, and constipation. If you have not entered menopause, surgery that removes both ovaries will cause menopause.

Menopause is the point in time at which you will not have another menstrual period again. When caused by surgery, the symptoms of menopause may be sudden and more severe. Symptoms of menopause include hot flashes, changes in mood, trouble sleeping, vaginal dryness, weight gain, and night sweats.

Cancer and recent abdominal surgery are also risk factors for developing blood clots, also known as deep vein thrombosis (DVT). Many patients are placed on blood thinners (either oral medications or injections) for up to 4 weeks after surgery to help prevent blood clots.

All of the side effects of ovarian cancer surgery are not listed here. Ask your treatment team for a full list of common and rare side effects. If a side effect bothers you, tell your treatment team. There may be ways to help you feel better.

The best advice that I could offer someone facing an illness is to stay positive no matter how much it tears you down, fight for the life you deserve, and please be pro-active because no one at any age, class, or race is invincible to cancer, disease, and illness."

– Christa
  Ovarian cancer survivor

Ovarian cancer stages

Cancer staging is the process of finding out how far the cancer has grown and spread in your body. The cancer stage is a rating of the extent of the cancer. Surgical staging is the most complete and accurate way to stage ovarian cancer. The information gained during surgery and surgical staging is used to determine the pathologic (post-surgery) stage.

The pathologic stage is based on the results of surgery and tests of tissue removed during surgery. The pathologic stage provides the most accurate picture of how far the cancer has spread. It is used to determine your treatment options after surgery.

A staging system is a standard way of describing the extent of cancer in the body. There are two staging systems for ovarian cancer: the American Joint Committee on Cancer (AJCC) staging system and the International Federation of Gynecology and Obstetrics (FIGO) staging system. These systems are very similar, but the FIGO system is used most often.

In the FIGO system, the cancer stage is defined by three main areas of cancer growth:

> - The extent of the first (primary) tumor

> - The spread of cancer to nearby lymph nodes

> - The spread of cancer to distant sites

Ovarian cancer stages are numbered from 1 to 4. The stages are also divided into smaller groups. This helps to describe the extent of cancer in more detail. The next section describes each cancer stage as defined by the FIGO staging system.

Ovarian cancers of the same stage tend to have a similar prognosis. A prognosis is the likely or expected course and outcome of a disease. In general, earlier cancer stages have better outcomes.

Other factors not used for cancer staging, such as your general health, are also very important. The FIGO stages of ovarian cancer are described next.

Stage 1

Cancer is only in one or both ovaries. Cancer has not spread to any other organs or tissues in the body.

Stage 1A

Cancer is in one ovary. The outer sac (capsule) of the ovary is intact. There is no cancer on the outside surface of the ovary. No cancer cells are found in ascites or washings.

Stage 1B

Cancer is in both ovaries. The capsules are intact and there is no cancer on the outside surface of the ovaries. No cancer cells are found in ascites or washings.

Stage 1C

Cancer is in one or both ovaries and one or more of the following has also happened:

> Stage 1C1 – The capsule of the ovary broke open (ruptured) during surgery. This is called surgical spill.

> Stage 1C2 – The capsule of the ovary ruptured before surgery, or there is cancer on the outer surface of the ovary or fallopian tube.

> Stage 1C3 – Cancer cells are found in ascites or washings.

Stage 1

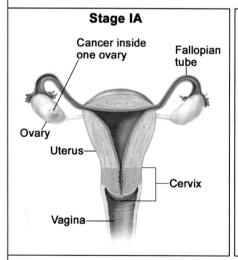

Stage IA
- Cancer inside one ovary
- Fallopian tube
- Ovary
- Uterus
- Cervix
- Vagina

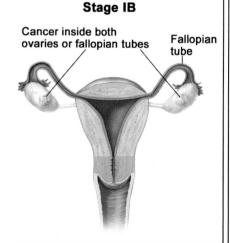

Stage IB
- Cancer inside both ovaries or fallopian tubes
- Fallopian tube

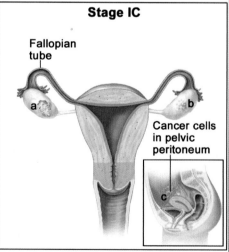

Stage IC
- Fallopian tube
- a
- b
- Cancer cells in pelvic peritoneum
- c

© 2010 Terese Winslow
U.S. Govt. has certain rights

Stage 2

Cancer is in one or both ovaries and has spread to other organs or tissues within the pelvis. Cancer has not spread outside the pelvis or to any lymph nodes.

Stage 2A

Cancer has grown into and/or spread implants on the uterus, fallopian tubes, ovaries, or all of these areas.

Stage 2B

Cancer has grown into and/or spread implants on other organs or tissues in the pelvis. This may include the bladder, sigmoid colon, rectum, or the peritoneum within the pelvis. The peritoneum is the tissue that lines the inside of the abdomen and pelvis and covers most organs in this space.

Stage 2

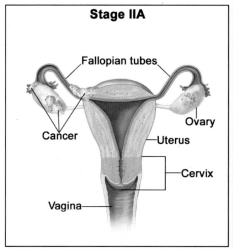
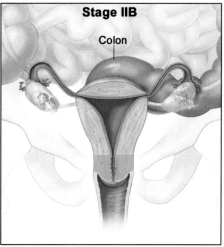

© 2011 Terese Winslow
U.S. Govt. has certain rights.

Stage 3

Cancer is in one or both ovaries. It has spread outside the pelvis to tissues in the belly (abdomen). And, one or both of the following has happened:

› Cancer has spread to the tissue lining the inside of the abdomen (peritoneum); or

› Cancer may have spread to lymph nodes in the back part of the abdomen behind the peritoneum.

Stage 3A1

Cancer has spread outside the pelvis, but only to lymph nodes in the back part of the abdomen—called retroperitoneal lymph nodes.

› Stage 3A1 (i) – Cancer in the lymph nodes is 10 mm (millimeters) or smaller.

› Stage 3A1 (ii) – Cancer in the lymph nodes is larger than 10 mm.

Stage 3A2

Cancer has spread to the tissue lining the abdomen, but it is so small it can only be seen with a microscope. Cancer may have also spread to lymph nodes in the back of the abdomen.

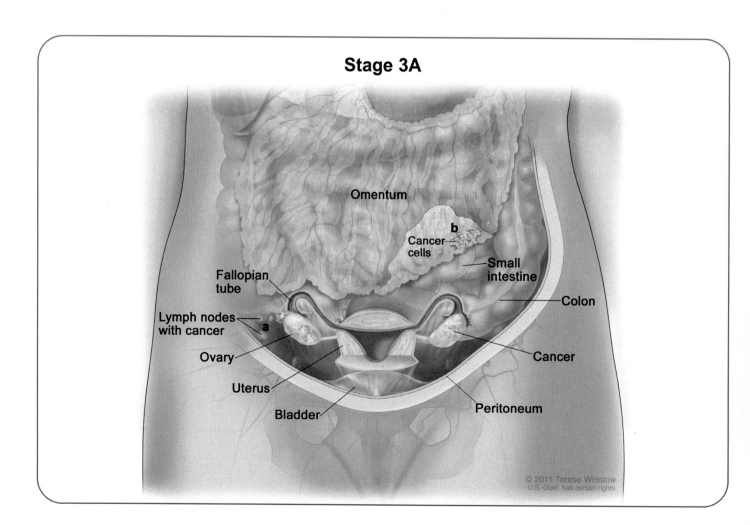

Stage 3A

© 2011 Terese Winslow
U.S. Govt. has certain rights

Stage 3B

Cancer has spread to the tissue lining the abdomen and it can be seen without a microscope. The areas of cancer spread are 2 cm (centimeters) or smaller. Cancer may have also spread to lymph nodes in the back of the abdomen.

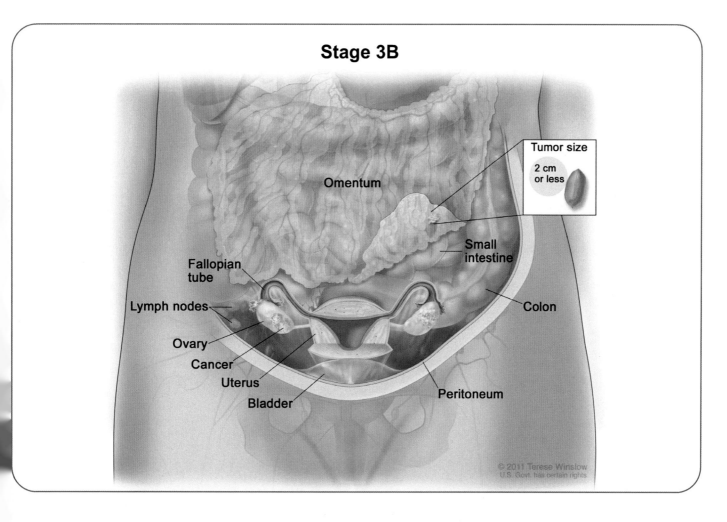

Stage 3B

Omentum

Tumor size

2 cm or less

Small intestine

Fallopian tube

Lymph nodes

Ovary

Cancer

Uterus

Bladder

Colon

Peritoneum

© 2011 Terese Winslow
U.S. Govt. has certain rights

Stage 3C

Cancer has spread to the tissue lining the abdomen and it can be seen without a microscope. The areas of cancer spread are larger than 2 cm. Cancer may have spread to lymph nodes in the back of the abdomen. It may have also spread to the outer surface of the liver or spleen.

Stage 4

Cancer has spread to other parts of the body, such as the liver, lungs, or brain. It may have spread to the inside of the liver or spleen. Cancer may have also spread to lymph nodes outside the abdomen—called distant lymph nodes.

Stage 4A

There are cancer cells in the fluid around the lungs. This is called pleural effusion. Cancer has not spread anywhere else outside the abdomen.

Stage 4B

Cancer has spread to the inside of the liver or spleen, to distant lymph nodes, or to other organs outside the abdomen.

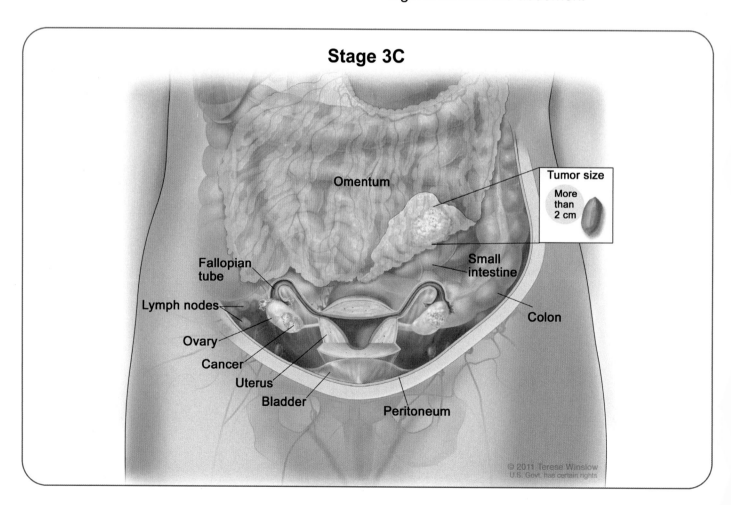

Stage 3C

Omentum

Tumor size
More than 2 cm

Fallopian tube

Small intestine

Lymph nodes

Ovary

Colon

Cancer

Uterus

Bladder

Peritoneum

© 2011 Terese Winslow
U.S. Govt. has certain rights

Stage 4

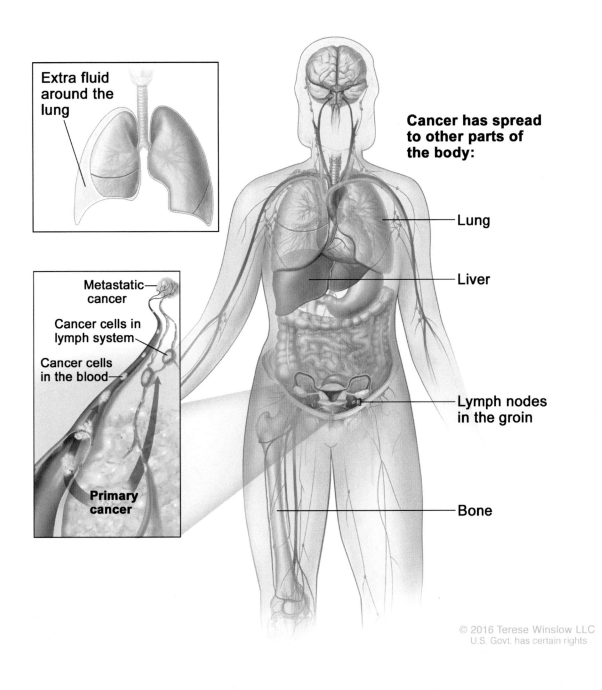

Extra fluid around the lung

Metastatic cancer

Cancer cells in lymph system

Cancer cells in the blood

Primary cancer

Cancer has spread to other parts of the body:

Lung

Liver

Lymph nodes in the groin

Bone

© 2016 Terese Winslow LLC
U.S. Govt. has certain rights

Chemotherapy after surgery

Chemotherapy is the use of medicine(s) to kill cancer cells. Chemotherapy drugs kill fast-growing cells throughout the body, including cancer cells and normal cells. When given after surgery, chemotherapy is known as adjuvant treatment. Your doctor may also refer to it as primary chemotherapy. Chemotherapy is a type of systemic therapy. The term systemic therapy is used to describe the fact that a medicine goes throughout the body or "system-wide."

Chemotherapy is recommended after surgery for **most** newly diagnosed stage I cancers. Observation may be an option for a stage IA or IB, grade 2 endometrioid tumor. Ask your doctor if this applies to your cancer. Chemotherapy is recommended after surgery for **all** newly diagnosed stage II, III, and IV ovarian cancers.

Platinum-based chemotherapy is recommended for ovarian cancer. As the name suggests, these chemotherapy medicines contain the metal platinum. Carboplatin, cisplatin, and oxaliplatin are platinum chemotherapy medicines. Carboplatin is the most commonly used of the three to treat ovarian cancer. A platinum agent is often combined with a different type of chemotherapy drug called a taxane to treat ovarian cancer. Paclitaxel and docetaxel are taxanes.

A targeted therapy called bevacizumab (Avastin®) may be added to chemotherapy after surgery for stage II, III, and IV ovarian cancers. Targeted therapy is treatment with drugs that target a specific or unique feature of cancer cells. These drugs stop the action of molecules that help cancer cells grow. Targeted therapy is less likely to harm normal cells than chemotherapy.

Bevacizumab is an angiogenesis inhibitor. Angiogenesis is the growth of new blood vessels. Like normal cells, cancer cells need the food and oxygen delivered in blood to live and grow. Cancer cells send out signals that cause new blood vessels to grow into the tumor to "feed" it. Bevacizumab blocks these signals so that new blood vessels will not form. As a result, the cancer cells do not receive the blood they need to live.

Currently recommended chemotherapy regimens for use after surgery are shown in Guide 1.

Guide 1
Chemotherapy regimens used after surgery

Paclitaxel and carboplatin

Paclitaxel, carboplatin, and bevacizumab (an option for stage II, III, or IV cancers)

Docetaxel and carboplatin

Carboplatin and liposomal doxorubicin

Carboplatin alone (a less harsh option for those over age 70 or who have other health problems)

Paclitaxel and cisplatin* (may be used for some stage II or III cancers)

This regimen involves both intravenous (IV) and intraperitoneal (IP) chemotherapy

Chemotherapy is given in cycles. A cycle includes days of treatment followed by days of rest. Giving chemotherapy in cycles lets the body have a chance to recover before the next treatment. The cycles vary in length depending on which drugs are used. Often, the cycles are 7, 14, 21, or 28 days long. The number of treatment days per cycle and the number of cycles given also vary depending on the regimen used.

For **stage I** cancers, at least 3 but up to 6 cycles are given. The number of chemotherapy cycles you receive depends on the tumor type and other features of your tumor. Six cycles of chemotherapy are recommended for high-grade serous tumors. Three to 6 cycles of chemotherapy are recommended for all other stage I tumor types. **For stage II, III, and IV cancers,** 6 cycles of chemotherapy are recommended.

The regimen that is best for you depends on a number of factors. This includes your age, overall health, and performance status—a rating of how well you are able to do daily activities. Another key factor is your risk for peripheral neuropathy—a nerve problem that causes pain, tingling, and numbness typically in the hands and feet. Neuropathy is a common side effect of paclitaxel and, to a lesser degree, carboplatin. If you have a high risk for nerve problems, then docetaxel and carboplatin may be a better option for you.

How chemotherapy is given
Most of the chemotherapy regimens for ovarian cancer are given intravenously, meaning the medicine is put directly into your bloodstream through a vein. This is called an IV infusion.

Chemotherapy can also be given as a liquid that is slowly injected into the abdomen (peritoneal cavity). This is called intraperitoneal (IP) chemotherapy. When given this way, higher doses of the drugs are delivered directly to the cancer cells in the belly area. IP chemotherapy is given through a thin tube called a catheter. The catheter is often placed inside the abdomen during surgery.

Monitoring during chemotherapy
During treatment, your doctor will monitor how well the chemotherapy is working and assess for side effects. The ways you may be monitored are listed below.

> A physical exam should be done every 1–3 cycles. A pelvic exam may also be done at the same time.

> CBC including measurement of platelet levels (as needed)

> Chemistry profile (as needed)

> Testing of CA-125 or other tumor markers (as needed prior to each cycle of chemotherapy)

> Imaging tests (as needed)

Side effects of chemotherapy

The side effects of chemotherapy depend on many factors, including the drug, the dose, and the person. In general, side effects are caused by the death of fast-growing cells, which are found in the intestines, mouth, and blood. As a result, common side effects include not feeling hungry, nausea, vomiting, mouth sores, hair loss, fatigue, low blood cell counts, increased risk of infection, bleeding or bruising easily, and nerve damage (neuropathy).

Some side effects are more likely or more severe when certain combination regimens are used. The docetaxel and carboplatin regimen is more likely to increase the risk of infection. The paclitaxel and carboplatin regimen is more likely to cause neuropathy. Neuropathy is a nerve problem that causes pain, tingling, and numbness in the hands and feet. Side effects also differ depending on how chemotherapy is given. IP chemotherapy tends to cause more severe side effects than IV chemotherapy. This includes infections, kidney damage, pain in the belly, and nerve damage.

Not all side effects of chemotherapy are listed here. Be sure to ask your treatment team for a full list of common and rare side effects of the drugs you receive. If a side effect bothers you, tell your treatment team. There may be ways to help you feel better.

Treatment response and next steps

Most **stage I** cancers do not need further treatment after chemotherapy. The next step is surveillance. See page 43.

For **stage II, III, and IV** cancers, the next step depends on how well chemotherapy worked. The possible outcomes of treatment are described next.

> A complete response means that there are no signs of cancer on imaging tests, a physical exam, or CA-125 blood tests after treatment.

> A partial response means that tests show a decrease in the amount of cancer, tumor size, or CA-125 levels. It means that the cancer improved, but is not completely gone.

> Stable disease is cancer that did not get better or worse during treatment.

> Progression means that the cancer continued to grow (progress) during or after treatment.

Complete or partial response

For many stage II, III, and IV cancers that have a complete or partial response to platinum-based chemotherapy, maintenance therapy is the next step. See the following page for information on maintenance therapy.

Stable disease or progression

If the cancer does not improve or gets worse, see *Persistent or recurrent cancer* on page 46.

Maintenance therapy

Maintenance therapy is the use of chemotherapy or targeted therapy after successful initial treatment for ovarian cancer. It can reduce the risk of cancer returning (recurrence) or extend the time until it returns or gets worse (progresses). Maintenance therapy is an option for stage II, III, and IV cancers that respond well or very well to surgery and platinum-based chemotherapy.

Your options for maintenance therapy depend on:

> Whether you have a *BRCA* mutation or are HRD positive

> Whether the chemotherapy regimen you were treated with included bevacizumab (Avastin®)

PARP inhibitors

Oral targeted therapies called PARP inhibitors are a newer option for maintenance therapy after initial treatment of ovarian cancer. Poly ADP-ribose polymerase (PARP) is an enzyme, or protein, that helps repair damaged DNA in cancer cells. Inhibiting, or blocking, PARP enzymes from fixing cancer cells damaged by chemotherapy allows the cancer cells to die. PARP inhibitors work best in HRD-positive cancers, which includes cancers caused by a *BRCA* mutation. These cancers have faulty DNA repair mechanisms, which leads to PARP enzymes stepping in to do the repairs. Blocking the PARP enzymes stops the repairs. Olaparib (Lynparza®) and niraparib (Zejula®) are PARP inhibitors currently used for maintenance therapy after initial treatment for ovarian cancer.

Side effects of PARP inhibitors
The most common side effects of PARP inhibitors are similar to those caused by chemotherapy and include fatigue, nausea, vomiting, and low blood cell counts. Rare but serious side effects include myelodysplastic syndrome (MDS) and acute myeloid leukemia (AML). MDS is a type of cancer in which the bone marrow does not make enough healthy blood cells and there are abnormal cells in the blood and/or bone marrow. AML is a fast-growing disease in which too many immature white blood cells are found in the bone marrow and blood. In some cases MDS can become AML.

Bevacizumab

Some chemotherapy regimens given after surgery include the targeted therapy bevacizumab (Avastin®). If you are a candidate for maintenance therapy, it means that chemotherapy that included bevacizumab worked well. In this case, bevacizumab can be given by itself as maintenance therapy. It may also be given in combination with a PARP inhibitor.

Determining your options

Bevacizumab was included in chemotherapy
If bevacizumab was included in the chemotherapy regimen you received after surgery and you have a *BRCA* mutation, combination maintenance therapy with both bevacizumab and the PARP inhibitor olaparib (Lynparza®) is recommended. While treatment with a PARP inhibitor alone (either olaparib or niraparib) is also an option, research suggests that bevacizumab and olaparib together may work better for people with a *BRCA* mutation.

If you do not have a *BRCA* mutation (or have not had a *BRCA* test), bevacizumab alone may be recommended for maintenance therapy. If you have had an HRD test and are HRD positive, combination therapy with both bevacizumab and olaparib (Lynparza) is recommended.

Bevacizumab was not included in chemotherapy
If bevacizumab was not included in the chemotherapy regimen you received after surgery and you have a *BRCA* mutation, maintenance therapy with either olaparib (Lynparza®) or niraparib (Zejula®) is recommended. Observation may be considered for some stage II cancers with a *BRCA* mutation.

If you do not have a *BRCA* mutation (or have not had a *BRCA* test), maintenance therapy with niraparib (Zejula®) may be an option, especially if you are HRD positive. Observation is also an option if you had a complete response to chemotherapy. A complete response means there are no signs of cancer in the body.

> There is not much research on maintenance therapy with a PARP inhibitor after initial treatment for patients with **stage II** ovarian cancer.
>
> If your cancer is stage II and you are eligible for maintenance therapy, talk to your doctor about your options.

How long does maintenance therapy last?
The length of maintenance therapy after initial treatment depends on the specific drug(s). Olaparib can be given for up to 24 months (2 years). Niraparib can be given for up to 36 months (3 years). When given with olaparib, bevacizumab can be given for up to 15 months. **However, any maintenance therapy will be stopped if one of the following occurs:**

> ➢ The cancer grows or spreads

> ➢ The side effects become intolerable or make it unsafe to continue

If surgery first is not an option

Having surgery first may not be an option because of the size and location of the tumor. Surgery first may also not be a good option if you are elderly, frail, have trouble doing daily activities, or have other serious health conditions. In this case, chemotherapy is given first to try to shrink the cancer before surgery. The medical name for this is neoadjuvant chemotherapy. It is important that a gynecologic oncologist is involved in making this treatment decision.

You will likely have a biopsy to confirm ovarian cancer before starting chemotherapy. If you have not yet had a referral for genetic risk evaluation and *BRCA1/2* testing, these may be ordered now.

Platinum-based chemotherapy is recommended. The same regimens used after surgery are also options for chemotherapy before surgery. See Guide 1 on page 37.

After a few cycles of chemotherapy, your doctor will check the status of the cancer to see how well chemotherapy worked and if surgery is an option. The goal of surgery is to remove as much of the cancer as possible, as well as the ovaries, fallopian tubes, and uterus. Surgery performed after chemotherapy is called interval debulking surgery (IDS).

For stage III disease, a chemotherapy technique called hyperthermic intraperitoneal chemotherapy (HIPEC) may be used during IDS. HIPEC is a newer technique in which a chemotherapy medicine called cisplatin is warmed and then put into the space between the organs of the abdomen during surgery.

If cancer **improves** after several cycles of chemotherapy, surgery is recommended. If cancer **stays the same**, your doctor may recommend proceeding with surgery or continuing chemotherapy to see if there is improvement. If there is, you would then have surgery. After surgery, you will have more chemotherapy followed by maintenance therapy. See page 40 for information on maintenance therapy.

If the cancer **grows or spreads (progresses)**, it is called persistent disease. Treatment for persistent cancer is similar to treatment for ovarian cancer that returns after treatment (recurrent cancer). See *Persistent or recurrent cancer* on page 46.

Surveillance

Surveillance begins when there are no signs of cancer after treatment. It is used to find early signs that cancer has come back.

When treatment is over, you should continue to see your cancer doctor on a regular basis. During the first two years after treatment, NCCN experts recommend you see your doctor every 2 to 4 months. During the following 3 years, the visits are spaced out to every 3 to 6 months. After that, one visit per year is recommended.

Many of the tests are only done on an as-needed basis. This means that your doctor will decide whether you need a particular test based on any symptoms you may have and other factors.

Genetic counseling is also recommended if it was not done before treatment. Genetic counseling is a discussion with a health expert about the risk for a disease caused by changes in genes. This is recommended because some health problems, including ovarian cancer, can run in families. It is important to know if you have any genetic mutations because you may be a candidate for certain newer targeted therapies.

The recommended follow-up schedule and the tests that may be used to monitor for the return of ovarian cancer are listed in Guide 2.

Guide 2 Follow-up care after treatment for all stages	
Schedule of follow-up visits	**First 2 years:** Every 2 to 4 months
	Next 3 years: Every 3 to 6 months
	After 5 years: Once a year
Follow-up tests and other care	Pelvic exam and physical exam
	Imaging of the chest, abdomen, and pelvis with CT, MRI, PET/CT or PET **(as needed)**
	CBC and blood chemistry profile **(as needed)**
	CA-125 blood test or other tumor markers **(if levels were high originally)**
	Referral for genetic risk evaluation **(if not already done)**
	Long-term wellness care

SNAPSHOT:
Hypersensitivity reactions

With repeat use of carboplatin and/or cisplatin, you are at an increased risk of having a hypersensitivity reaction (also called an allergic reaction) that could be life-threatening. If your treatment team hasn't brought it up, below are some questions you can ask to get more information about this risk.

• How likely is it that I will have an allergic reaction to chemotherapy?

• How will I know if I'm having an allergic reaction? What are the symptoms?

• Does the staff on hand know how to manage hypersensitivity reactions?

• Will the right medical equipment be available in case I have an allergic reaction?

Recurrence

The return of cancer after treatment is called a recurrence, or a relapse. Your doctor may suspect that cancer has returned if:

> Your CA-125 levels are going up

> Cancer was found on follow-up imaging tests

> You have symptoms of ovarian cancer, such as pain or bloating in your pelvis or belly, unexplained weight loss, upset stomach, constipation, trouble eating or feeling full fast, fatigue, and needing to urinate often or urgently

If recurrence is suspected or confirmed, additional testing will be done to gather more information. If you haven't had imaging tests recently, you may have them now. This may include a CT, MRI, PET, or PET/CT scan of your chest, abdomen, and pelvis.

If you have not already been tested for the following biomarkers, you should be tested now:

> *BRCA1* and *BRCA2* mutations

> Microsatellite instability/mismatch repair (MSI/MMR)

Other biomarkers your doctor may test for to help guide treatment include:

> Homologous recombination deficiency (HRD)

> *NTRK* gene fusions

> Tumor mutational burden (TMB)

See page 17 for more information on the biomarkers listed above.

You didn't have chemotherapy

If your CA-125 levels are rising or you have symptoms of recurrence and you did not yet have chemotherapy, the cancer is treated the same as if you were newly diagnosed. This means that you will have surgery to remove the cancer followed by chemotherapy. The type and extent of surgery depends on how far the cancer has spread.

You had chemotherapy

If your CA-125 levels are going up but there are no other signs of recurrence, treatment does not need to be started right away. It is safe to wait until you have symptoms or other signs of recurrence. Starting treatment immediately does not always lead to better outcomes.

In some cases, however, your doctor may prefer not to delay treatment. See the next section, *Persistent or recurrent cancer*.

My cancer experience has been a journey of self awareness. Along the way, I have met some inspiring women who have enriched my life. As I reach my 30th year of survivorship, I realize that hope and love sustained me through those early dark days. There is no such thing as false hope; we are all entitled to hope; hope that tomorrow will be a better day. And, of course, the love of family and friends."

– Risa
Ovarian cancer survivor

Persistent or recurrent cancer

Everyone with persistent or recurrent ovarian cancer is encouraged to consider enrolling in a clinical trial for treatment. Treatment with a newly developed investigational drug or combination of drugs may provide benefit.

Supportive care is an option for everyone with ovarian cancer, whether you are in active treatment or not. Supportive care can help relieve the symptoms of cancer and the side effects of treatment. It aims to relieve discomfort and improve quality of life.

Platinum-resistant cancer

Ovarian cancer is referred to as "platinum-resistant" if:

> It does not improve or gets worse during platinum-based chemotherapy

> It returns less than 6 months after successful treatment with platinum-based chemotherapy

Because platinum-based chemotherapy drugs like cisplatin and carboplatin did not work very well against the cancer, a different type of drug is recommended for recurrence treatment. There are many non–platinum-based chemotherapy regimens that may be used. Talk to your doctor about which is right for you.

Other options for systemic therapy may include a PARP inhibitor, hormone therapy, targeted therapy, and immunotherapy. These are described in more detail on the next page. You should talk to your doctor about any clinical trials you may be eligible for at this time.

Platinum-sensitive ovarian cancer

If you enter complete remission after platinum-based chemotherapy and cancer returns more than 6 months later, the cancer is considered "platinum-sensitive." This means that platinum-based chemotherapy drugs work well against the cancer.

Because it worked well initially, platinum-based chemotherapy is typically recommended for recurrent platinum-sensitive disease, especially if it is the first recurrence. The targeted therapy bevacizumab may be added to chemotherapy. Your doctor may want to do surgery to remove all visible cancer before beginning recurrence treatment. This is called cytoreductive surgery.

If you have a complete or partial response to platinum-based recurrence chemotherapy, maintenance therapy is an option. If bevacizumab was included in your recurrence chemotherapy regimen, it can be continued as maintenance therapy. If you have not already been treated with a PARP inhibitor, maintenance therapy with a PARP inhibitor may be an option, and is recommended for patients with a *BRCA* mutation. See page 40 for more information on PARP inhibitors. After successful chemotherapy for recurrent cancer, maintenance therapy with a PARP inhibitor can be continued until one of the following occurs:

> The cancer grows or spreads

> The side effects become intolerable or make it unsafe to continue

Other options for recurrence treatment therapy may include a PARP inhibitor, hormone therapy, targeted therapy, and immunotherapy. These are described in more detail below. The targeted therapy entrectinib is an option for *NTRK* gene fusion-positive tumors.

Depending on the specific recurrence treatment planned, radiation therapy may also be given to help with symptoms. More information is provided below.

Other options for recurrence treatment

PARP inhibitor
A PARP inhibitor may be an option for recurrence treatment if you have already received at least 2 lines of chemotherapy and have a *BRCA* mutation or are HRD positive. Niraparib, olaparib, and rucaparib are PARP inhibitors used for recurrence therapy.

Other options for recurrence therapy may include hormone therapy, targeted therapy, and immunotherapy. The targeted therapies larotrectinib and entrectinib are options for *NTRK* gene fusion-positive tumors.

Immunotherapy

The immune system is your body's natural defense against infection and disease. Immunotherapy increases the activity of your immune system. By doing so, it improves your body's ability to find and destroy cancer cells. An immunotherapy drug called pembrolizumab (Keytruda®) may be used to treat recurrent ovarian cancer. It is an immune checkpoint inhibitor. It may be an option if your cancer is MSI-H/dMMR or has a high tumor mutational burden. See page 17 for more information on these biomarkers.

For more information on the side effects of immune checkpoint inhibitors, see the NCCN Guidelines for Patients *Immunotherapy Side Effects: Immune Checkpoint Inhibitors* at NCCN.org/patientguidelines.

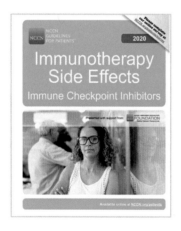

Endocrine therapy

Estrogen and progesterone are hormones made by the ovaries. They help some ovarian cancers grow. Some patients are prescribed hormones after they become menopausal to help with symptoms of menopause, such as hot flashes. This treatment with hormones, known as hormonal replacement therapy or "HRT," may help some cancers grow. In some cases treatment can be used to block these hormones from working, or to lower hormone levels, in order to help slow ovarian cancer growth. This is called endocrine therapy or anti-estrogen therapy. This therapy may be used for persistent or recurrent ovarian cancer.

Different types of endocrine therapy drugs work in different ways. These drugs that may be used for ovarian cancer include:

> Tamoxifen stops the effect of estrogen on cancer cell growth. It is in a class of drugs called antiestrogens.

> Anastrozole, exemestane, and letrozole lower estrogen levels in the body. They are in a class of drugs called aromatase inhibitors.

> Leuprolide acetate causes the ovaries to make less estrogen and progesterone. It is in a class of drugs called luteinizing hormone-releasing hormone (LHRH) agonists.

> Megestrol acetate stops the effect of estrogen on cancer cell growth. It is in a class of drugs called progestins.

Endocrine therapy can cause a number of side effects. Symptoms of menopause are common. Such symptoms include hot flashes, changes in mood, vaginal dryness, trouble sleeping, and night sweats. Other common side effects of hormone therapy are vaginal discharge, weight gain, swelling in the hands and feet, fatigue, and less interest in sex. Blood clots are a rare but serious side effect of tamoxifen. Aromatase inhibitors can weaken your bones and may also cause joint and muscle pain.

Radiation therapy to help with symptoms

Depending on the specific recurrence treatment planned, radiation therapy may also be given to help with symptoms. This is known as palliative radiation therapy. Radiation treatment to the pelvis can cause the vagina to become shorter and narrower. This is called vaginal stenosis. Vaginal stenosis can make it uncomfortable or even painful to have sex, or to have vaginal examinations by a doctor. Vaginal dilator therapy can be used to prevent or treat vaginal stenosis. A vaginal dilator is a device used to gradually stretch or widen the vagina. You can start using a dilator as soon as 2 to 4 weeks after radiation therapy has ended. You can continue to use it for as long as you want.

Survivorship

Cancer survivorship begins on the day you learn you have ovarian cancer. Survivorship focuses on the physical, emotional, and financial issues unique to cancer survivors. Managing the long-term side effects of cancer and its treatment, staying connected with your primary care doctor, and living a healthy lifestyle are important parts of survivorship.

For many survivors, the end of active treatment signals a time of celebration but also of great anxiety. This is a very normal response. You may need support to address issues that arise from not having regular visits with your cancer care team. In addition, your treatment plan should include a schedule of follow-up cancer tests, treatment of long-term side effects, and care of your general health.

Your primary care doctor

After finishing cancer treatment, your primary care doctor will play an important role in your care. Your cancer doctor and primary doctor should work together to make sure you get the follow-up care you need. Your oncologist should develop a survivorship care plan that includes:

> A summary of your cancer treatment history

> A description of possible late- and long-term side effects

> Recommendations for monitoring for the return of cancer

> Information on when your care will be transferred to your primary care physician. The plan should also outline specific responsibilities for both your cancer doctor and your primary care physician

> Recommendations on your overall health and well-being

Healthy habits

It is important to keep up with other aspects of your health. There are a few steps you can take that will make a big difference in your overall health, including:

> Getting screened for other types of cancer. Your primary care doctor should tell you what cancer screening tests you should have based on your gender, age, and risk level.

> Getting other recommended health care for your age, such as blood pressure screening, hepatitis C screening, and immunizations (such as the flu shot).

> Maintaining a healthy body weight by exercising at a moderate intensity for at least 30 minutes most days of the week.

> Eating a healthy diet with lots of plant-based foods and drinking little to no alcohol.

> If you are a smoker, quit! Your treatment team will be able to provide you with (or direct you to) resources on quitting smoking.

More information

For more information on cancer survivorship see *NCCN Guidelines for Patients: Survivorship Care for Healthy Living* and *Survivorship Care for Cancer-Related Late and Long-Term Effects* at NCCN.org/patientguidelines.

These resources address many topics relevant to survivors of ovarian cancer, including:

> Anxiety, depression, and distress

> Cognitive dysfunction

> Fatigue

> Pain

> Sexual dysfunction

> Sleep disorders

> Healthy lifestyles

> Immunizations

> Employment, insurance, and disability concerns

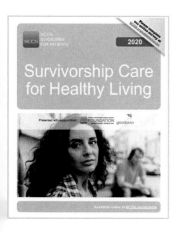

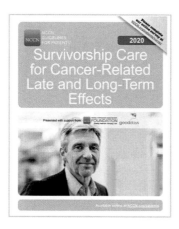

Key points

- Surgery is the recommended first treatment for ovarian cancer whenever possible. Ovarian cancer surgery should be performed by a gynecologic oncologist.

- Surgery for ovarian cancer usually involves removing both ovaries, both fallopian tubes, the uterus, and the cervix.

- Fertility-sparing surgery (described below) may be an option for some women with very early ovarian cancer that has not spread beyond the ovaries.

- Ovarian cancer is staged during surgery to remove the cancer— called surgical staging.

- Platinum-based chemotherapy is recommended after surgery for most stage I cancers and for all stage II, III, and IV ovarian cancers.

- A targeted therapy called bevacizumab may be added to chemotherapy for stage II, III, and IV ovarian cancers.

- Most stage I cancers do not need further treatment after chemotherapy.

- Maintenance therapy is recommended for many stage II, III, and IV cancers that show a complete or partial response to initial treatment.

- Maintenance therapy can reduce the risk of cancer returning (recurrence) or extend the time until it returns or gets worse (progresses).

- Oral targeted therapies called PARP inhibitors are a newer option for maintenance therapy after initial treatment of ovarian cancer.

- PARP inhibitors work best in cancers with a *BRCA* mutation and/or HRD-positive cancers.

- Bevacizumab may be used alone or in combination with a PARP inhibitor for maintenance therapy if it was included in chemotherapy.

- Survivorship focuses on the physical, emotional, and financial issues unique to cancer survivors.

3
Making treatment decisions

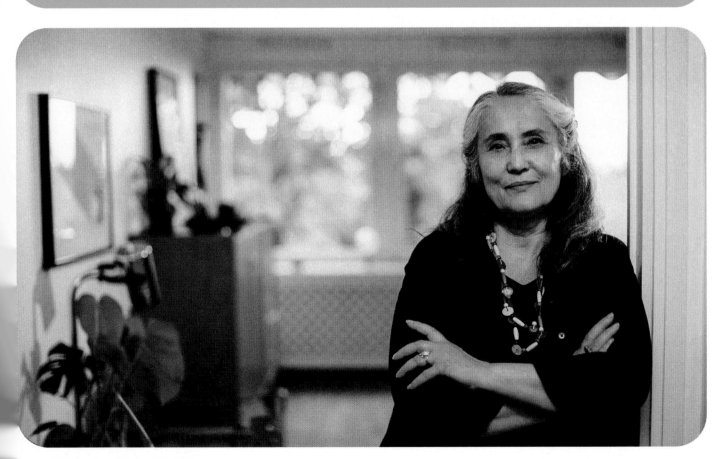

It is important to be comfortable with the cancer treatment you choose. This choice starts with having an open and honest conversation with your doctor.

It's your choice

In shared decision-making, you and your doctors share information, discuss the options, and agree on a treatment plan. It starts with an open and honest conversation between you and your doctor.

Treatment decisions are very personal. What is important to you may not be important to someone else.

Some things that may play a role in your decision-making:

> What you want and how that might differ from what others want

> Your religious and spiritual beliefs

> Your feelings about certain treatments like surgery or chemotherapy

> Your feelings about pain or side effects such as nausea and vomiting

> Cost of treatment, travel to treatment centers, and time away from work

> Quality of life and length of life

> How active you are and the activities that are important to you

Think about what you want from treatment. Discuss openly the risks and benefits of specific treatments and procedures. Weigh options and share concerns with your doctor. If you take the time to build a relationship with your doctor, it

will help you feel supported when considering options and making treatment decisions.

Second opinion

It is normal to want to start treatment as soon as possible. While cancer can't be ignored, there is time to have another doctor review your test results and suggest a treatment plan. This is called getting a second opinion, and it's a normal part of cancer care. Even doctors get second opinions!

Things you can do to prepare:

> Check with your insurance company about its rules on second opinions. There may be out-of-pocket costs to see doctors who are not part of your insurance plan.

> Make plans to have copies of all your records sent to the doctor you will see for your second opinion.

Support groups

Many people diagnosed with cancer find support groups to be helpful. Support groups often include people at different stages of treatment. Some people may be newly diagnosed, while others may be finished with treatment. If your hospital or community doesn't have support groups for people with cancer, check out the websites listed in this book.

Questions to ask your doctors

Possible questions to ask your doctors are listed on the following pages. Feel free to use these or come up with your own. Be clear about your goals for treatment and find out what to expect from treatment. Keep a notebook handy to record answers to your questions.

Questions to ask your doctors about testing

1. What tests will I have?

2. Where will the tests take place? Will I have to go to the hospital?

3. How long will it take? Will I be awake?

4. Will any test hurt?

5. What are the risks?

6. How do I prepare for testing?

7. Should I bring a list of my medications?

8. Should I bring someone with me?

9. How soon will I know the test results?

10. Who will explain the test results to me?

11. Can I have a copy of the test results and pathology report?

12. Who will talk with me about the next steps? When?

Questions to ask your doctors about treatment

1. What treatments do you recommend?

2. Will I have more than one treatment?

3. What are the risks and benefits of each treatment? What about side effects?

4. Will my age, general health, and other factors affect my treatment choices?

5. Do you have a clinical trial available for me? (also see next page)

6. Would you help me get a second opinion?

7. How soon should I start treatment? How long does treatment take?

8. Where will I be treated? Will I have to stay in the hospital or can I go home after each treatment?

9. What can I do to prepare for treatment?

10. What symptoms should I look out for during treatment?

11. How much will the treatment cost? How can I find out how much my insurance company will cover?

12. How likely is it that I'll be cancer-free after treatment?

13. What is the chance that the cancer will come back?

14. Are there supportive services that I can get involved in? Support groups?

Questions to ask your doctors about clinical trials

1. What clinical trial is right for me?

2. What is the purpose of the study?

3. How many people will be in the clinical trial?

4. What are the tests and treatments for this study? How often will they occur?

5. Has the treatment been used before? Has it been used for other types of cancers?

6. What side effects can I expect from the treatment? Can the side effects be controlled?

7. How long will I be in the clinical trial?

8. Will I be able to get other treatment if this treatment doesn't work?

9. How will you know the treatment is working?

10. Who will help me understand the costs of the clinical trial?

What is your experience?

1. Are you board-certified? If yes, in what area?

2. How many patients like me have you treated?

3. How many procedures like the one you're suggesting have you done?

4. Is this treatment a major part of your practice?

5. How many of your patients have had complications?

Websites

American Cancer Society
cancer.org/cancer/ovarian-cancer.html

Cancer.net
cancer.net/cancer-types/ovarian-fallopian-tube-and-peritoneal-cancer

FORCE: Facing Our Risk of Cancer Empowered
facingourrisk.org

National Cancer Institute
cancer.gov/types/ovarian

National Ovarian Cancer Coalition
ovarian.org

NormaLeah Ovarian Cancer Institute
normaleah.org

Ovarcome
ovarcome.org

Ovarian & Breast Cancer Alliance of Washington State
knowthesymptoms.org

Ovarian Cancer Research Alliance
ocrahope.org

Sharsheret
sharsheret.org

Unite for HER
uniteforher.org

U.S. National Library of Medicine Clinical Trials Database
clinicaltrials.gov

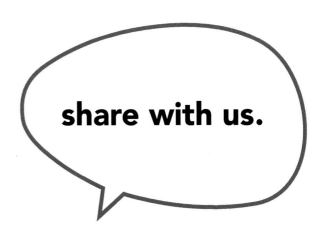

share with us.

Take our survey
And help make the
NCCN Guidelines for Patients
better for everyone!

NCCN.org/patients/comments

Words to know

abdomen
The belly area between the chest and pelvis.

adjuvant treatment
Treatment given after the main treatment used to rid the body of disease.

ascites
Abnormal fluid buildup in the belly (abdomen) or pelvis.

bilateral salpingo-oophorectomy (BSO)
Surgery to remove both ovaries and both fallopian tubes.

biopsy
Removal of small amounts of tissue from the body to be tested for disease.

blood chemistry profile
A test that measures the amounts of many different chemicals in a sample of blood.

***BRCA1* or *BRCA2* genes**
Genes involved in DNA repair. Abnormal changes (mutations) of either of these genes increases the risk of developing breast and ovarian cancer.

cancer antigen 125 (CA-125)
A substance that may be found in high amounts in the blood of patients with ovarian cancer. CA-125 levels may also help monitor how well cancer treatments are working or if cancer has come back.

cancer grade
A rating of how much the cancer cells look like normal cells.

cancer stage
A rating of the growth and spread of cancer in the body.

cancer staging
The process of rating and describing the extent of cancer in the body.

capsule
A thin layer of tissue that surrounds an organ—like the skin of an apple.

carcinoembryonic antigen (CEA)
A substance that may be found in the blood of people who have certain cancers or who smoke tobacco. CEA levels may help keep track of how well cancer treatments are working or if cancer has come back. A type of tumor marker.

cervix
The lower part of the uterus that connects to the vagina.

chemotherapy
Drugs that kill fast-growing cells throughout the body, including normal cells and cancer cells.

chest x-ray
A test that uses x-rays to make pictures of the inside of the chest.

clear cell carcinoma of the ovary
A rare type of epithelial ovarian cancer, in which the insides of the cells look clear when viewed under a microscope. A less common ovarian cancer (LCOC).

clinical trial
Research on a test or treatment to assess its safety or how well it works.

combination regimen
The use of two or more drugs.

complete blood count (CBC)
A test of the number of blood cells.

complete response
All signs and symptoms of cancer are gone after treatment.

completion surgery
Surgery to remove the remaining ovary, fallopian tube, uterus, and all cancer that can be seen.

computed tomography (CT) scan
A test that uses x-rays from many angles to make a picture of the inside of the body.

contrast
A substance put into your body to make clearer pictures during imaging tests.

cytoreductive surgery
Surgery to remove as much cancer as possible. Also called debulking surgery.

debulking surgery
Surgery to remove as much cancer as possible. Also called cytoreductive surgery.

endometrioid carcinoma of the ovary
A type of epithelial ovarian cancer. Grade 2 and 3 endometrioid tumors are common. Grade 1 endometrioid tumors are less common ovarian cancers (LCOCs).

epithelial cells
Cells that form the outer layer of tissue around organs in the body.

epithelial ovarian cancer
Cancer that starts in the cells that form the outer layer of tissue around the ovaries.

fallopian tube
A thin tube through which an egg travels from the ovary to the uterus.

fertility-sparing surgery
Surgery that only removes one ovary and fallopian tube so that a woman can still have babies.

gastrointestinal (GI) evaluation
A test to view the organs that food passes through when you eat.

gastrointestinal tract
The group of organs that food passes through when you eat.

general anesthesia
A controlled loss of wakefulness from drugs.

genetic counseling
A discussion with a health expert about the risk for a disease caused by changes in genes.

genetic counselor
A health expert that has special training to help patients understand changes in genes that are related to disease.

genetic testing
Tests to look for changes in coded instructions (genes) that increase the risk for a disease.

germ cell
Reproductive cells that become eggs in women and sperm in men.

gynecologic oncologist
A surgeon who is an expert in cancers that start in a woman's reproductive organs.

hereditary ovarian cancer
Ovarian cancer caused by abnormal coded information in cells that is passed down from parent to child.

hormone
Chemicals in the body that activate cells or organs.

hot flashes
A health condition of intense body heat and sweat for short periods.

hyperthermic intraperitoneal chemotherapy (HIPEC)
A cancer treatment that involves filling the abdominal cavity with warmed chemotherapy drugs.

hysterectomy
Surgery to remove the uterus.

implant
Cancer cells that broke away from the first tumor and formed new tumors on the surface of nearby organs and tissues.

infusion
A method of giving drugs slowly through a needle into a vein.

intraperitoneal (IP) chemotherapy
Chemotherapy drugs given directly into the belly (abdomen) through a small tube.

intravenous (IV) chemotherapy
Chemotherapy drugs given through a needle or tube inserted into a vein.

invasive implant
Cancer cells that broke away from the first tumor and are growing into (invading) supporting tissue of nearby organs.

lactate dehydrogenase (LDH)
One of a group of enzymes found in the blood and other body tissues, and involved in energy production in cells. An increased amount in the blood may be a sign of tissue damage and some types of cancer or other diseases.

laparotomy
Surgery with a long, up-and-down cut through the wall of the belly (abdomen).

less common ovarian cancers (LCOC)
Rare types of ovarian cancer, some of which are epithelial cancers. Includes carcinosarcoma, clear cell carcinoma, mucinous carcinoma, grade 1 endometrioid, low-grade serous, borderline epithelial, malignant sex-cord stromal, and malignant germ cell tumors. Also called less common ovarian histologies (LCOHs).

liver function test
A blood test that measures chemicals that are made or processed by the liver to check how well the liver is working.

low malignant potential (LMP) tumor
A tumor formed by abnormal cells that start in the epithelial cells of the ovary. This tumor type is slow growing and does not invade other tissue. A less common ovarian cancer (LCOC). Also called a borderline epithelial tumor.

lymph
A clear fluid containing white blood cells that fight infection and disease.

lymph nodes
Small groups of special disease-fighting cells located throughout the body.

lymph vessels
Small tubes that carry lymph—a clear fluid with white blood cells that fight infection and disease—throughout the body.

Lynch syndrome
Abnormal changes within genes that increase the chances of developing colon, rectal, endometrial, ovarian, and other cancers. It is also called hereditary non-polyposis colorectal cancer (HNPCC).

magnetic resonance imaging (MRI) scan
A test that uses radio waves and powerful magnets to make pictures of the inside of the body.

maintenance treatment
Treatment given to continue (maintain) good results of prior treatment.

medical oncologist
A doctor who is an expert in treating cancer with drugs such as chemotherapy.

menopause
The point in time when menstrual periods end.

menstrual cycle
Changes in the womb and ovaries that prepare a woman's body for pregnancy.

metastasis
The spread of cancer cells from the first tumor to another body part.

microscopic metastases
Cancer cells that have spread from the first tumor to another body part and are too small to be seen with the naked eye.

mucinous carcinoma of the ovary
One of 4 types of epithelial cancer. A less common ovarian cancer (LCOC).

mutation
An abnormal change in the instructions in cells for making and controlling cells.

neuropathy
A nerve problem that causes pain, tingling, and numbness in the hands and feet.

noninvasive implant
Cancer cells that broke away from the first tumor and are growing on the surface of nearby organs, but are not growing into (invading) tissue.

observation
A period of testing to watch for cancer growth.

omentum
The layer of fatty tissue that covers organs in the belly (abdomen).

ovary
One of a pair of organs that make hormones and eggs for reproduction.

pathologist
A doctor who is an expert in testing cells and tissue to find disease.

pelvic exam
A physical exam of the vagina, cervix, uterus, fallopian tubes, and ovaries.

pelvis
The area of the body between the hip bones.

peritoneal cavity
The space inside the belly (abdomen) that contains abdominal organs such as the intestines, stomach, and liver.

peritoneal washing
A test in which a special liquid is used to wash the inside of the belly (peritoneal cavity) to check for cancer cells.

peritoneum
The layer of tissue that lines the inside of the belly (abdomen) and pelvis and covers most organs in this space.

persistent disease
Cancer that stayed the same—didn't get better or worse—during treatment.

platinum agent
A cancer drug that is made with platinum. These drugs damage DNA in cells, which stops them from making new cells and causes them to die.

platinum-based chemotherapy
Treatment with two or more chemotherapy drugs and the main drug is made with platinum. Such drugs include cisplatin and carboplatin.

platinum-resistant
When cancer drugs made with platinum, such as cisplatin and carboplatin, do not work well against the cancer.

platinum-sensitive
When cancer drugs made with platinum, such as cisplatin and carboplatin, work well against the cancer.

poly (ADP-ribose) polymerase (PARP) inhibitor
A type of targeted therapy that blocks a protein in cells called PARP that helps repair damaged DNA.

positron emission tomography (PET)
A test that uses a sugar radiotracer and x-rays from many angles to view the shape and function of organs and tissues inside the body.

primary tumor
The first mass of cancer cells in the body.

prognosis
The likely or expected course and outcome of a disease.

radiologist
A doctor who is an expert in interpreting imaging tests.

recurrence
The return of cancer after treatment. Also called a relapse.

recurrence treatment
Treatment that is given after prior treatments failed to kill all the cancer or keep it away.

regimen
A treatment plan that specifies the drug(s), dose, schedule, and length of treatment.

relapse
The return of cancer after treatment. Also called a recurrence.

reproductive system
The group of organs that work together for reproduction. In women, this includes the ovaries, fallopian tubes, uterus, cervix, and vagina.

serous
A type of epithelial ovarian cancer. Grade 2 and 3 (high-grade) serous tumors are the most common ovarian cancers. Grade 1 (low-grade) serous tumors are less common ovarian cancers (LCOCs).

sugar radiotracer
A form of sugar that is put into your body and lets off a small amount of energy that is absorbed by active cells.

supportive care
Treatment given to relieve the symptoms of a disease. Also called palliative care.

surgical staging
The process of finding out how far cancer has spread by performing tests and procedures during surgery to remove the cancer.

targeted therapy
Treatment with drugs that target a specific or unique feature of cancer cells.

taxane
A type of cancer drug that blocks certain cell parts to stop a cell from dividing into two cells.

treatment response
An outcome or improvement related to treatment.

tumor
An abnormal mass formed by the overgrowth of cells.

tumor marker
A substance found in body tissue or fluid that may be a sign of cancer.

ultrasound
A test that uses sound waves to take pictures of the inside of the body.

unilateral salpingo-oophorectomy (USO)
Surgery that removes one ovary and the attached fallopian tube.

uterus
The organ in the pelvis where a fetus grows and develops during pregnancy. Also called womb.

vagina
The hollow, muscular tube through which babies are born.

vein
A blood vessel that carries blood back to the heart from all parts of the body.

washings
Sample of liquid that is tested for cancer cells after it is used to "wash" the inside of the belly (peritoneal cavity).

white blood cell
A type of blood cell that helps fight infections in the body.

NCCN Contributors

This patient guide is based on the NCCN Clinical Practice Guidelines in Oncology (NCCN Guidelines®) for Ovarian Cancer, Version 1.2021. It was adapted, reviewed, and published with help from the following people:

Dorothy A. Shead, MS
Senior Director
Patient Information Operations

Rachael Clarke
Senior Medical Copyeditor

Tanya Fischer, MEd, MSLIS
Medical Writer

Laura J. Hanisch, PsyD
Medical Writer/Patient Information Specialist

Stephanie Helbling, MPH, MCHES®
Medical Writer

Susan Kidney
Graphic Design Specialist

John Murphy
Medical Writer

Erin Vidic, MA
Medical Writer

Kim Williams
Creative Services Manager

NCCN Clinical Practice Guidelines in Oncology (NCCN Guidelines®) for Ovarian Cancer, Version 1.2021 were developed by the following NCCN Panel Members:

Deborah K. Armstrong, MD/Chair
The Sidney Kimmel Comprehensive Cancer Center at Johns Hopkins

Ronald D. Alvarez, MD, MBA/Vice Chair
Vanderbilt-Ingram Cancer Center

Jamie N. Bakkum-Gamez, MD
Mayo Clinic Cancer Center

Lisa Barroilhet, MD
University of Wisconsin Carbone Cancer Center

Kian Behbakht, MD
University of Colorado Cancer Center

*Andrew Berchuck, MD
Duke Cancer Institute

Lee-may Chen, MD
UCSF Helen Diller Family Comprehensive Cancer Center

Mihaela Cristea, MD
City of Hope National Medical Center

*Marie DeRosa, RN

Eric L. Eisenhauer, MD
Massachusetts General Hospital Cancer Center

David M. Gershenson, MD
The University of Texas MD Anderson Cancer Center

Heidi J. Gray, MD
Fred Hutchinson Cancer Research Center/Seattle Cancer Care Alliance

Rachel Grisham, MD
Memorial Sloan Kettering Cancer Center

Ardeshir Hakam, MD
Moffitt Cancer Center

Angela Jain, MD
Fox Chase Cancer Center

Amer Karam, MD
Stanford Cancer Institute

Gottfried E. Konecny, MD
UCLA Jonsson Comprehensive Cancer Center

Charles A. Leath III, MD
O'Neal Comprehensive Cancer Center at UAB

Joyce Liu, MD, MPH
Dana-Farber/Brigham and Women's Cancer Center

Haider Mahdi, MD, MPH
Case Comprehensive Cancer Center/University Hospitals Seidman Cancer Center and Cleveland Clinic Taussig Cancer Institute

Lainie Martin, MD
Abramson Cancer Center at the University of Pennsylvania

Daniela Matei, MD
Robert H. Lurie Comprehensive Cancer Center of Northwestern University

Michael McHale, MD
UC San Diego Moores Cancer Center

Karen McLean, MD, PhD
University of Michigan Rogel Cancer Center

David S. Miller, MD
UT Southwestern Simmons Comprehensive Cancer Center

David M. O'Malley, MD
The Ohio State University Comprehensive Cancer Center - James Cancer Hospital and Solove Research Institute

Sanja Percac-Lima, MD, PhD
Massachusetts General Hospital Cancer Center

Iena Ratner, MD
Yale Cancer Center/Smilow Cancer Hospital

Steven W. Remmenga, MD
Fred & Pamela Buffett Cancer Center

Roberto Vargas, MD
Case Comprehensive Cancer Center/University Hospitals Seidman Cancer Center and Cleveland Clinic Taussig Cancer Institute

*Theresa L. Werner, MD
Huntsman Cancer Institute at the University of Utah

Emese Zsiros, MD, PhD
Roswell Park Comprehensive Cancer Center

NCCN Staff

Jennifer Burns
Manager, Guidelines Support

Anita Engh, PhD
Oncology Scientist/Medical Writer

* Reviewed this patient guide. For disclosures, visit NCCN.org/disclosures.

NCCN Cancer Centers

Abramson Cancer Center
at the University of Pennsylvania
Philadelphia, Pennsylvania
800.789.7366 • pennmedicine.org/cancer

Fred & Pamela Buffett Cancer Center
Omaha, Nebraska
402.559.5600 • unmc.edu/cancercenter

Case Comprehensive Cancer Center/
University Hospitals Seidman Cancer
Center and Cleveland Clinic Taussig
Cancer Institute
Cleveland, Ohio
800.641.2422 • UH Seidman Cancer Center
uhhospitals.org/services/cancer-services
866.223.8100 • CC Taussig Cancer Institute
my.clevelandclinic.org/departments/cancer
216.844.8797 • Case CCC
case.edu/cancer

City of Hope National Medical Center
Los Angeles, California
800.826.4673 • cityofhope.org

Dana-Farber/Brigham and
Women's Cancer Center |
Massachusetts General Hospital
Cancer Center
Boston, Massachusetts
617.732.5500
youhaveus.org
617.726.5130
massgeneral.org/cancer-center

Duke Cancer Institute
Durham, North Carolina
888.275.3853 • dukecancerinstitute.org

Fox Chase Cancer Center
Philadelphia, Pennsylvania
888.369.2427 • foxchase.org

Huntsman Cancer Institute
at the University of Utah
Salt Lake City, Utah
800.824.2073
huntsmancancer.org

Fred Hutchinson Cancer
Research Center/Seattle
Cancer Care Alliance
Seattle, Washington
206.606.7222 • seattlecca.org
206.667.5000 • fredhutch.org

The Sidney Kimmel Comprehensive
Cancer Center at Johns Hopkins
Baltimore, Maryland
410.955.8964
www.hopkinskimmelcancercenter.org

Robert H. Lurie Comprehensive
Cancer Center of Northwestern
University
Chicago, Illinois
866.587.4322 • cancer.northwestern.edu

Mayo Clinic Cancer Center
Phoenix/Scottsdale, Arizona
Jacksonville, Florida
Rochester, Minnesota
480.301.8000 • Arizona
904.953.0853 • Florida
507.538.3270 • Minnesota
mayoclinic.org/cancercenter

Memorial Sloan Kettering
Cancer Center
New York, New York
800.525.2225 • mskcc.org

Moffitt Cancer Center
Tampa, Florida
888.663.3488 • moffitt.org

The Ohio State University
Comprehensive Cancer Center -
James Cancer Hospital and
Solove Research Institute
Columbus, Ohio
800.293.5066 • cancer.osu.edu

O'Neal Comprehensive
Cancer Center at UAB
Birmingham, Alabama
800.822.0933 • uab.edu/onealcancercenter

Roswell Park Comprehensive
Cancer Center
Buffalo, New York
877.275.7724 • roswellpark.org

Siteman Cancer Center at Barnes-
Jewish Hospital and Washington
University School of Medicine
St. Louis, Missouri
800.600.3606 • siteman.wustl.edu

St. Jude Children's Research Hospital/
The University of Tennessee
Health Science Center
Memphis, Tennessee
866.278.5833 • stjude.org
901.448.5500 • uthsc.edu

Stanford Cancer Institute
Stanford, California
877.668.7535 • cancer.stanford.edu

UC Davis
Comprehensive Cancer Center
Sacramento, California
916.734.5959 | 800.770.9261
health.ucdavis.edu/cancer

UC San Diego Moores Cancer Center
La Jolla, California
858.822.6100 • cancer.ucsd.edu

UCLA Jonsson
Comprehensive Cancer Center
Los Angeles, California
310.825.5268 • cancer.ucla.edu

UCSF Helen Diller Family
Comprehensive Cancer Center
San Francisco, California
800.689.8273 • cancer.ucsf.edu

University of Colorado Cancer Center
Aurora, Colorado
720.848.0300 • coloradocancercenter.org

University of Michigan
Rogel Cancer Center
Ann Arbor, Michigan
800.865.1125 • rogelcancercenter.org

The University of Texas
MD Anderson Cancer Center
Houston, Texas
844.269.5922 • mdanderson.org

University of Wisconsin
Carbone Cancer Center
Madison, Wisconsin
608.265.1700 • uwhealth.org/cancer

UT Southwestern Simmons
Comprehensive Cancer Center
Dallas, Texas
214.648.3111 • utsouthwestern.edu/simmons

Vanderbilt-Ingram Cancer Center
Nashville, Tennessee
877.936.8422 • vicc.org

Yale Cancer Center/
Smilow Cancer Hospital
New Haven, Connecticut
855.4.SMILOW • yalecancercenter.org

Index

Made in the USA
Middletown, DE
02 July 2021